Sex after 50 -

Fact or Fiction?

elven

Sex after 50 – Fact or Fiction?

Changing Beliefs about Aging and Intimacy

Ditte Trolle

elven

Sex after 50 – Fact or Fiction? Changing Beliefs about Aging and Intimacy.

Copyright © 2014 by Ditte Trolle.

ISBN 978-87-995480-2-6

This is a revised version of "Sex efter 50 – om kærlighed, krop og kultur i en moden alder", published by Elven in 2012. This version is published by Elven 2014.
Contact: trolle@elven.dk

Cover: Daliborka Mijailovic

Disclaimer

All contents in this book are for general information purposes only and not intended or implied to be a substitute for any kind of advice, medical or other. Any person in need for this kind of service should consult a professional adviser. If you have or suspect you may have a health problem, please consult your health care provider.

Even if the author has made great efforts to ensure that the contents in this book are correct, errors and imperfections may occur. Neither the publisher, nor the author will accept any responsibility for damages or losses occurring as a result of using this book.

Unless otherwise specified, the views in this book are my own and a result of my cultural viewpoint, being a Scandinavian woman. Nothing included or said in this book is meant to offend anyone in any way. If this ever happens to be the case, I wish to apologize for the incident.

Contents

Introduction

Imagine an elderly couple taking a walk together, holding hands. What thoughts and feelings come to mind? Most people probably have similar thoughts: It looks wonderful; it's a scene displaying tenderness and love. They are still fond of each other and they support each other in their old age. You may feel moved and think that you, too, would like that kind of relationship when you grow old. It would probably not offend you if the two old lovers gave each other a kiss in public, as long as it's small and quick, without too much close body contact.

But if you're like the majority of people, there's a limit to your enthusiasm and tolerance. For instance, try bringing up the topic of sex and people over 50 with a teenager and you will probably get a look of distrust and disgust. And this reaction is not exclusive to teenagers; it tends to be the attitude of the majority of the younger generations until they themselves approach the age of 50 and begin to speculate about the future of their erotic lives, perhaps already noticing some changes. Even though the older generations are growing in numbers almost worldwide, most still have nowhere to go to find information and inspiration about sexuality in the third age of life. The subject is taboo, resulting in disapproval and silence.

So if the elderly couple you are watching decides to give each other a long, wet kiss in public or touch each other in a way that could lead to thoughts of a passionate encounter between them, it may very well be perceived as ridiculous, inappropriate and offensive. It is as if it is impossible to imagine that sex can be an important part of life for people over the age of 50.

Older people and sex are incompatible. An elderly man or woman who makes an obvious effort to be sexually attractive is not considered a possible erotic partner or an admirable role model, but just an embarrassing old fool. An elderly man who is preoccupied with sex will, at most, qualify for the term "dirty old man", while an elderly woman who sends erotic signals is so unthinkable that there isn't even a derogatory term for her.

Advertising targeted at young people is filled with bare skin and sexual innuendo. This is never the case when the target audience is older people. The entire advertising industry is firmly focused on youth, and this certainly helps to cement the perception that youth is the happiest and most important period in life, also when it comes to sex. That's what it's all about, and it is in the early years that we experience all essential experiences in life - including sex.

When Viagra became available in 1998, the negative view of sex and seniority became very clear in the media, particularly in the U.S. Older people should not be preoccupied with the physical aspects of love. It was inappropriate and unacceptable. Viagra would transform dignified old men into horny, impatient thugs who chased young women without inhibition in order to have sex with them, day and night. No one really considered how Viagra would affect the lives of older women, except perhaps the women themselves, who did not openly comment much on the subject.

The Greek-American writer and columnist Arianna Huffington is one woman who has clearly expressed her opinion about the elderly and sex. What prompted her was Senator Bob Dole, who at the age of 75 signed a deal with Pfizer to appear in advertisements for Viagra. He was seriously chastised in a column by Huffington, who accused him of having "completely lost a sense of the stages of life". Apparently, when you're 75, there should be more important things on your mind than your libido. She claimed it was about time he became a little less self-centered and went on to suggest that, instead, he might start building houses for the poor.

So even in our relatively liberal society sex does not really sell tickets if the parties are over 50. But where does this opinion derive from? Why shouldn't people over 50 have sex and enjoy it, and why would anybody even feel provoked by it? There are at least three possible explanations for this.

The first is advocated by people who call upon the order of nature. In their eyes sex is not something you just do for fun. It is an activity meant to achieve pregnancy and have children, and consequently should only be practiced by heterosexuals of childbearing age. For others, such as older people, gays, and lesbians, sex is an activity in conflict with nature and should thus be banned. This of course affects mainly women, who can only become pregnant for a limited part of their lives. However, the way people live and behave today generally differs greatly from the "order of nature", and the proportion of sexual encounters for the sole purpose of procreation is probably very small. Most people do in fact have sex just for fun. So why wouldn't the elderly?

The next explanation is actually the exact opposite of the first one. Rather than following nature, it dictates that we ought to disassociate ourselves from it. We are not animals with uncontrollable urges, but humans who should be noble, dignified and in full control of our passions. Sex is associated not only with tenderness and love, but also with vigor, strength, and power, with the shedding of all inhibitions. And people approaching old age should not have anything to do with such things. As an appropriate transition to a possible life after death, they ought to spend their remaining years in a rocking chair, their minds focused on reflection and spiritual interests.

Perhaps this explains why it is particularly difficult to imagine one's parents as sexually active, a thought that can make most people cringe and very quickly try to think of something else. This is particularly true in young people who are only just discovering their own sexuality. In several forums online, children from ten years of age and up complain about being able to hear their parents making love on the other side of the bedroom wall. They think it's embarrassing, awkward and sometimes even scary. The typical comment is: "It's ok that they did it once, when they were going to have me - but that's it!"

Few young people wish their parents to have a good sex life, and very few seem to have a positive attitude towards their parent's sexuality. Perhaps it scares them to imagine their mother and father consumed by passion. Children depend on their parents and want them to be composed and sane and prepared to take care of their children's needs, and maybe they perceive it as a threat to imagine their caretakers occupied with something clearly so important, but impossible to understand.

There is generally a great psychological resistance to imagining family members in sexual situations. This goes both ways; it's just as repulsive for parents to think of their children having sex as the other way around. The reason is probably that parents, siblings and other close relatives are sexually taboo, so placing them in sexual scenarios, however imagined, is tantamount to incest.

Finally, there is the view of sex as being so strongly linked to beauty that sex between old people simply becomes too unattractive and ugly. As a rule, sex implies some degree of nudity and enjoyment of the naked body, and the body is only attractive when it is young and beautiful. Countless films, books and music throughout the ages are based on the mixture of youth, beauty and sex. Youth itself is attractive.

But why is that? Why do we perceive youth as beautiful and attractive? Well, probably a very simple but important biological mechanism is at work here. The ability to have children is greatest in the years just after puberty and decreases steadily as the years go by, particularly for women. So when we see a young, slender body with the right proportions - hourglass shape for women, broad shoulders and slim hips for men - and we find that person attractive, it is most likely nothing more than a reaction in our reptilian brain, which is ruled by primitive responses - survival of the individual and reproduction of the species. This part of the brain registers a body shape suggesting a normal hormonal balance and fertility, good health and strength as appropriate for an uncomplicated pregnancy and the ability to take care of new generations of small reptiles.

So when sex is seen as a natural activity for young people, the only reason may be that young people are the best suited to have children.

The logical consequence of this argumentation is, of course, that sex is unnatural for the elderly. It is strange that we are so highly evolved and yet our thoughts and opinions are still so strongly guided by biology and the importance of reproduction. What about all the other things, the feelings that make us want entice a partner into bed? What about intimacy, sensuality, desire, pleasure and closeness? Are these emotions stronger and more important for young people than for older people?

No – fortunately they're not, quite the contrary. Sexuality seems to change character with age. While rough and very physical sex may be what you look for while you're young, the softer sides of sex take over as you grow older.

So there are several possible reasons why so little is said about elderly sexuality. But here comes the good news for those of you who are under 50: you have something to really look forward to. Even if they may adopt a low-key approach to it, the elderly also have active sex lives that give them pleasure and gratification. In fact, more and more research shows that both the desire and the ability to have sex continue after the childbearing years, and that although older people's sex lives often differ from those of young people, they experience just as much joy and fulfillment – maybe even more.

Agnes, Age 75

Some believe that life ends at 40. That's when it begins! That's when you know who you are. Sex is just as delightful for me now as when I was younger, but I don't want to have sex all night. I have a good friend, who has been my lover for over 25 years. We don't live together, but we always have a good time together. He's a little younger than I am.

I have osteoarthritis and that makes it a little difficult to move about as much as I'd like to, but I get by. I had a hip replacement two years ago, and that was really a good thing. In the beginning, you may only flex the hip 90 degrees, and it takes some time before you figure out how to have sex. You have to be a little creative and try different positions. If you can't do that then I think you haven't gotten enough out of life. If it hurts, you just have to try another position.

Nobody talks about older people and sex.

I've never had any problems apart from a bit of vaginal dryness. I use hormones in my vagina and a lubricant. I don't really notice that I'm dry; for me, the feeling is the same. It may take a little longer now to reach orgasm, and I don't have more than one, but the feeling is the same as when I was younger. Also it doesn't matter now if we don't have sex as often, it doesn't have to be every day. But the desire is still there, and I also masturbate once in a while when I feel like it.

I don't understand women who've lost the desire for sex. When I was younger, I could have sex all the time. Now my friend and I don't throw ourselves at each other the moment we get inside the door, we sit together a little first, enjoying each other's company.

Sometimes one of us gets more pleasure out of sex than the other, which is fine, too. And he needs a little help from time to time. That's the way it is with men.

He had a heart attack once, and in the beginning we were a little nervous, will this work out okay? ... But he was told at the hospital that he could have sex if he wanted to. He had to ask about it, though. Doctors should remember to tell you what you can do, not just what you can't do.

Sex is healthy. People who have sex feel younger inside and don't grow old as fast as others. My brother is 71 and has been a widower for ten years. He now has a new girlfriend, who is a widow. There is sex in that relationship too.

Sex in Old Age - Fundamentals

A hundred years ago, it was considered harmful or even perverse to have a sex life if you were a senior citizen. If it did happen, the general attitude in society was to conceal or ridicule it. Mature couples with a desire for each other felt ashamed embarrassed and abnormal. What would their children say if they suspected that their old parents had an active sex life?

Sex was not openly talked about, and the great variation in how people express their sexuality was unknown to the general public. However, in the 1900s, attitudes toward sex slowly began to change, and around 1950 the American biologist Alfred Kinsey published his reports on human sexuality: the first one about men, the second about women. Over 10,000 Americans had responded to questions about how often and in what ways they had sex; about homosexuality, sexual fantasies, sexual positions; about how much they made use of foreplay and many other aspects of their sex lives.

But only one percent of the women Kinsey dealt with in his report were over the age of 60 and almost no one was over 80. Older men were slightly better represented, but it is still quite striking: Kinsey's research has had a major impact on the understanding of sexuality and broke many taboos, but with regard to the elderly, his views were not particularly progressive nor did they differ from the prevailing views in society. Older people were irrelevant when it came to sex.

Since then, there has been significant improvement. In recent years, an abundance of research reports have shed light on the sex lives of older people. Approaches to the subject have been medical, psychological, sociological and anthropological, but the reports share a couple of significant problems that make it difficult to compare them: There is no consensus on the definition of sexual activity, nor is there agreement on what age is considered old.

Defining Sex

"I did not have sexual relations with that woman," said President Bill Clinton, waving his finger on live television after his close encounters with Monica Lewinsky. In court he argued that she just gave him blowjobs and that he himself remained passive. Thus, he did not believe this could be defined as a sexual relationship. That he chose to present this line of argument at all shows that there is room for doubt about how to define sexual activity. In deeply conservative Christian circles in the United States, young people are not allowed to have sex before marriage, and they circumvent this prohibition by enjoying all sorts of erotic variants except vaginal intercourse.

However, in my part of the world a blowjob is definitely a sexual relationship, and nobody would agree with Clinton. Neither did Mrs. Clinton, who for a period of time after the impeachment forbade him access to their shared bedroom. The president himself was probably never in doubt that he was having a sexual experience, and the same presumably applies to Ms. Lewinsky, although she apparently did not get much more out of it than the dubious honor and a few drops of presidential semen on her blue dress.

Here in Northern Europe, most people would agree that in addition to intercourse with a penis in a vagina, anal sex and oral sex are also sexual acts. These are all activities that require at least two participants and involve genital contact. Masturbation, with or without vibrators, dildos and other toys, is also defined as sex.

In the case against Clinton, sexual relations were defined as: "A person engages in sexual relations when the person knowingly engages in or causes contact with the genitalia, anus, groin, breast, inner thigh, or buttocks of any person with the intent to arouse or gratify the sexual desire of any person." But do the genitals have to be involved at all? There are lots of other areas on the body where touch can cause arousal and make you desire sex. A kiss on the lips, for instance; is that sex, or are we now talking about something better described as erotic physical contact? And what about sexual thoughts, fantasies and sexy talk, such as phone sex or sex chatting on the Internet? There is no physical contact, but it is still a sexual activity.

Everyone has probably been in a situation where the intentions of another person were unclear. Was that just a friendly hug? Or is he up to something else? Is she just a cheerful woman, or is that sparkle in her eye inviting me to go a little further?

If you are unable to sense the signals or to interpret them correctly, you can be terribly mistaken about a situation, and misunderstandings can occur with serious consequences for both yourself and others. The ultimate risk is rape, if a man does not understand that a women's no actually means no. Or accusations of sexual harassment when an overly friendly boss thinks he is just spreading a cozy and informal atmosphere at the office.

Finding a definition of sexual activity that we can all agree on doesn't seem that simple. Many words circle around the phenomenon without being clear-cut. A lot of emotions and sensations are associated with sex – delight, lust, intimacy, closeness, passion, pleasure, satisfaction, desire, sensuality, arousal, just to mention a few of the positive ones. However, sex can take place without any of these present, and so pain, disgust, impatience, unhappiness, boredom, anger and animosity can also be associated with sex. Yet we may have a common understanding of sex as a certain sensation stemming from the fact that everyone who has once experienced the physical sensations triggered by sexual activity will later recognize the same sensations as being sexual in nature.

In situations where the law is involved, there is a need for concepts that are precise and unambiguous, so you would suppose that it is possible to find a definition of sexual activity in jurisprudence to be used in connection with accusations of sexual abuse. Unfortunately you can't. Danish law defines sexual harassment as "unwanted and offensive acts of a sexual nature". We won't get much closer than that.

Does this really have anything to do with sexuality at a mature age? Yes, it does. If you want to find facts about how often older people are sexually active, you have to define exactly what is meant by the term "sexual activity" in order to ask the right questions. In the vast majority of the existing research, the term is not adequately defined or only defined as ordinary vaginal intercourse, and in addition to the presupposition that all couples are heterosexual, this also does not cover what many elderly people perceive as having a sex life.

Many studies show that sexual intercourse is not crucial to older people. All forms of intimate physical contact are valuable and understood as erotic. Kissing and hugging, being close together, feeling each other's bodies and recognizing each other's scent, fondling each other, giving and receiving oral sex all belong to the sex lives of the elderly.

So does masturbation, although it is particularly difficult to collect information on this specific subject. Older people are very reluctant to talk about it, and in surveys the questions about masturbation often remain unanswered. Apparently this is a strong taboo. Many older people have grown up in a society where masturbation was not only subject to shame and guilt, but was also believed to be harmful. It was thought that masturbation led to weakness and moral decay and could even cause blindness and the mysterious condition called spinal cord decay – feared by many young people in the earlier times, but never seen in real life, as far as I know.

Defining Old Age

How old do you have to be to be defined as "elderly" in research on older people's sex lives? Well, that depends on who you ask. If you ask young people around the age of 20, "old" may very well be over 40, and a lot of researchers on sexuality seem to be of the same opinion. A global study of the sex lives of the elderly from 2006 included people aged 40 to 80 years. In a study from Hong Kong of the sexuality of Chinese citizens, not one single woman over 50 is included.

When a researcher is planning a scientific study, the study design will inevitably be influenced by the prejudice of the researcher and her preconceived understanding of the state of things. It is impossible to think 100 percent out of the box. The researcher has carefully considered, and probably discussed with any co-workers, the maximum age limit of the respondents she could include in her study without offending anyone. Maybe sex is so unthinkable over a certain age that it would be too embarrassing to ask about it? What about people's personal boundaries and sense of decency?

In fact, embarrassment seems to be entirely the questioner's personal issue. Older people don't mind being asked, as long as it is done respectfully and the setting feels safe and inspires confidence. So there is no reason for researchers or doctors to feel reluctant to ask older people about their sexual problems or to provide information about how disease and treatment affect their sexuality.

There are, however, other obstacles to obtaining information. Many researchers have been confronted with the fact that younger relatives of the elderly don't like the idea of bringing the sex lives of their loved ones into focus. The young and middle-aged may find it taboo-breaking and unacceptable to suggest that their old parents' interest in each other is anything but purely platonic. Again, what is crucial here is not consideration for the elderly, but rather the reluctance of the younger generations to think of their parents as sexual beings.

If you want to conduct research on the sex lives of older generations, there are other things you have to take into account as well – things that don't matter as much to younger generations. Older people's lives differ in many ways from those of younger people. Looks, the appearance of the body, are not as important anymore, while the body's capability may be pivotal, as illness and disabilities become more prevalent and play a bigger role the older you get.

Furthermore, whether you live alone or in a relationship also matters. With advancing age, more and more people lose their partners, particularly heterosexual women. Their partners are often slightly older than themselves, and a woman's life expectancy is still several years longer than a man's. For a single woman of 75, it's not all that easy to find a new partner. You don't just go to a bar on Friday night and hope to meet somebody nice and attractive. You don't make new friends as easily as you did in your 20s, and when it comes to men of the same age, the selection generally tends to thin out a little.

Researchers investigating sexuality in old age may choose either to show a snapshot or describe trends over time. Perceptions of the mature sex life, both those of the older people themselves and of society in general, evolve in line with other changes in society and culture. Those who are now 70 years old were in their 20s when the sexual revolution started to take off in the mid-sixties. Sexual liberation has had its influence on them and their attitudes toward sex are probably quite different than those of their parents.

Sex and Aging Around the World

At intervals of about 25 years – in 1976 and 2000 - researchers interviewed Swedish 70 year olds about their sexuality. The study focused on the frequency of intercourse, the general importance of sex and sexual satisfaction. There appeared to be a clear change over the years. In 1976, only 25 percent of men thought that sex contributed positively to their quality of life. In 2000, practically all men thought so, and for women, the change was even greater. The proportion who considered sex a joy in life increased from five to 78 percent. Virtually none of the respondents distanced themselves from the idea that older people can have be sexually active.

During the 25 years between the reports, the proportion of 70-year-old men who indicated had had intercourse during the preceding year rose from 50 to 66 percent. Women also experienced an increase, although only half as many of the 70-year-old women indicated they had had intercourse. Only one in ten of the sexually active 70 year olds considered their sex lives to be unsatisfactory.

Scandinavia is not at all unique in this field. A similar study was conducted in the U.S., but instead of examining how attitudes to sex have changed over time, different age groups between the ages of 57 and 85 were compared. And sexual activity was not confined to intercourse but included all kinds of sexual practice. The study found that older Americans are almost as sexually active as older Swedes.

Both studies show that especially when you're not quite young anymore, having a regular partner means a lot for your opportunity to be sexually active. In this area, the circumstances of life differ considerably for men and women. The difference becomes greater the higher up in the age groups you get: In their 50s, almost as many women as men have a partner, whereas in their 80s far more women than men live alone. In the youngest age bracket, 60 percent of the women are sexually active, while in the oldest, only 20 percent are. But those who do have sex have it regularly, usually several times a month.

However, many of those interviewed also talk about problems: Many women suffer from lack of desire, vaginal dryness and problems with achieving orgasm. Many men have difficulties becoming erect and also with climaxing. But while men experience increasing problems with age, this does not apply to women. A woman who has a good and rewarding sex life when she is past menopause has very good chances that she will continue to have that also in her old age.

This comes as a surprise to most. My old friend Marianne, for instance, said with a smile at the age of 62: "It has really taken me by surprise that sex could be so fantastic at my age. I would never have imagined that! When I was younger, I thought it would be over by now."

So there appears to be good cause to be happy about the quality of the sexual lives of the older generations in the western world, particularly in Scandinavia. Elsewhere, it is less positive. A comprehensive international report on the sexual well-being of older people in 29 different countries showed surprisingly large differences between the continents. In this study, "elderly" was defined as people over 40. Participants in the study answered questions about their physical and emotional satisfaction with their sex lives; about how well functioning they felt their sex lives were; and how important sex was to them.

The responses showed that women in general were more dissatisfied than men. In addition, the study found clear geographical differences: respondents from the western part of the world gave their sex lives the highest rating, but did not consider sex a pivotal factor in life. In the Muslim world, sex was perceived as very important, but generally less satisfactory. Moreover, the difference between men's and women's satisfaction was high, with women by far the most dissatisfied group.

The last group consisted entirely of Asian countries, and here there is truly cause for concern: In Japan, only 27 percent of men and 12 percent of women over 40 felt that sex was important. This is a very notable difference from the 70-year-old Swedes, where the vast majority felt that sex contributed positively to their quality of life. And the few times the Japanese engaged in some activity between the sheets, they didn't find it particularly rewarding: Only 18 percent of men and ten percent of women felt that sex gave them any physical satisfaction.

In Hong Kong, not even one third of Chinese men are sexually active after the age of 65, and almost everyone has erectile issues.

When searching research report databases like MEDLINE for studies on aphrodisiacs, agents that allegedly strengthen the desire and ability to have sex (rhinoceros horn powder and the like), it is striking how many of the author names originate in Asia. In the light of the number of negative reports on sexuality in East Asia, this is certainly no coincidence.

But in the West, things look brighter. Even older people living in nursing homes are still interested in sex, and if they are able to get it, they think it makes them feel good. They have a positive attitude toward sex and would like to have it if possible, but they are also very good at keeping their expectations realistic.

Expectations may not always be good when you live in a nursing home. A Danish thesis from 2011 on how nurses handle the sexuality of nursing home residents indicates that nurses find it difficult to talk to the elderly about sex and are afraid that they will offend the elderly by bringing the matter up. Moreover, an older couple who move into a nursing home may not be given the possibility to sleep together at all.

This is certainly going to change. There is growing recognition that sex is important in all stages of life. In the U.K. there are now guidelines for nursing home staff on how to deal with residents' sexuality, respect their individual life stories and their choices in sexual matters, and the issue is also on the agenda in many other places throughout the world.

But although the need for sex does not disappear with age, older people seem to be able to regulate their needs better than younger people do. If they lack a partner, or if disease has made it difficult or impossible to have sex, they put up with it, block out the desire and don't miss it. A non-existent sex life doesn't bother the elderly as much as it does younger people, who in a similar situation feel deprived, frustrated and suffer from poor self-esteem.

As long as the older people's views on sex are the same as the prevailing views in the community they live in – that it's not something they should expect to have – they may just be humbly satisfied with whatever they can get.

Jens, Age 79

I'll be 80 soon. I have been married to the same woman for 56 years and engaged for 59. During all these years, our sex life hasn't changed at all. Well, maybe it doesn't happen as often as before. I would say that we make love about eight-ten times a month. It works just as well as it always has done and it is still just as fantastic for both of us as it always has been, also for my wife. She is 77 and still ravishing, to me at least – a tall slim girl.

We are healthy and fit, both of us. My legs aren't quite what they used to be, so I use a walker and a cane. But I exercise my back at home every day and I also do pelvic floor exercises. I also like training on my bike, and twice a week my wife and I go to a gym together.

Two years ago I had an operation for rectal cancer. I was lucky and they were able to remove all of it, so I didn't need any radiation or chemotherapy. After that, we didn't have sex for three months. But we lay in each other's arms, kissed, had a good time and sensed the comfort. And we talked about how if things were to stay that way, we wouldn't have any problems with it. But then suddenly, in the middle of the day, I had an erection again. "Looks like it's ready to go again", I said, and now our sex life is exactly the same as it always has been.

I think it used to be more or less taken for granted that old people didn't have a sex life. And I know that many of my friends, who are the same age I am, don't do it anymore. It was like that with my parents-in-law. Not that we spoke openly about it. It was just assumed between the lines, you know. If it happens because one half of a couple loses the desire, it's a loss for the other half, and my father-in law missed it a lot. My mother-in-law told him that is was all right if he found someone else to have sex with, as long as he didn't tell her about it. I think that quite a lot of couples make that deal.

In our family we can talk about sex, and our children know very well that we have a wonderful intimate life together. Not that we sit and talk dirty, mind you, but there are some joking remarks. And a few years ago my grandchild asked me: "Tell me, Grandpa, do you make love with Grandma?" And then we had a little chat about that.

If I were to give tips on how to maintain a good sex life when you get older, I would say that it's important to be considerate. You have to keep yourself healthy, be clean, be very careful with your hygiene. But above all you have to be very good to each other; there must be a feeling of security and comfort. We never fall asleep at night without giving each other a kiss, and we never get up in the morning without lying close for a few moments, kissing each other. And then sometimes, you know, one thing leads to another.

Sex and Culture

According to research, sex is regarded as much more pleasant in some parts of the world while less so in others. Why is it that older men in Stockholm are satisfied with their sex lives, but in Shanghai they're unhappy? Why do women in Europe want to continue to be sexually active as long as possible, while women in Japan apparently want to quit - the sooner the better? Are Asians simply less interested in sex than Europeans? Or just generally more dissatisfied? Why does the quality of older people's sex lives differ so much between generations and different parts of the world?

It's hard to believe that the differences are genetic, inherited over the generations. It's been shown that today's 70-year-old Swedes have more sex and are more satisfied with it than just a generation ago, and genes simply do not change that quickly. So that leaves us with the environment we are brought up in, the culture that imprints on us our values and beliefs about what's good and bad in life.

Culture teaches us what's worth striving for and what's not important; what is good and bad behavior in ourselves and in others. The biology of our bodies enables us to feel desire and respond to it, but culture determines how we react to desire and how we manage it. The views on the sex lives of older people are affected by the perceptions of sex in general in our culture. They are also influenced by the general opinion of older people, and of the conduct and lifestyles that are considered appropriate for them.

And when it comes to sex, society's rules for acceptable behavior are much stricter for women than for men. This applies to women of all ages, including those over 50.

Forbidden Desires

Gunilla was a girl at my school. She was a few years older than me. She did not hide the fact that she thought sex was great and wonderful. Measured by the standards of the time, she was extremely advanced and accessible, and without hesitating too long, she went to bed with the boys she fancied. It was an unforgivable social misstep. She was soon regarded as the whore of the school, the other girls whispered behind her back, and when she was admitted to hospital with gonorrhea, everybody agreed that she had it coming. She should never have exposed her desire in that shameless way. She was, of course, never invited to the parties held by the respectable girls and boys.

That was the way it was in the fifties in the town in northern Sweden where I grew up. At that time, Sweden was branded worldwide as a country of free sex, and sexual equality between men and women was part of the Swedish democratic model. There was sexual education in schools, there were bare breasts in the movies and contraceptives could be bought without restrictions. But in reality, the liberalistic agendas did not change people's minds and hearts as quickly as they were put down on paper. Gunilla's story is just one example of how women had to handle things carefully and quietly when it came to sex.

Another example was the dress code for pregnant women. A woman expecting a baby could in no way send any sexual signals or show off her body. A virtuous thing, such as a pleated tent with a little white collar, was appropriate. Breast-feeding in public was, of course, out of the question. It was generally taken for granted that women were well-behaved, controlled and non-provocative in every way.

This basic assumption has left a strong imprint not only on our knowledge of sexuality, but also, for instance, on our knowledge of women's drinking habits of 50 years ago. There was no research on this, as it was not considered appropriate to ask women about alcohol at that time, thus insinuating that there were women who were not able to control themselves and live according to society's rules.

There were other rules for men. It was considered quite normal that men were subject to their desires and urges, and they were allowed to follow them. In sexual education classes children were taught that it was a man's nature to be sexually aggressive and it was a woman's duty to hold back. So when Gunilla was condemned and reviled for her behavior, it was perfectly in line with current standards.

The sexual revolution in the sixties completely transformed the concept of sexual morals. Both men and women were allowed sexual freedom. Showing your breasts or being completely naked on the beach was okay, as was living together and even having children without being married. Some Danish communes had special rooms for making love, and it was not a requirement that there was only one couple at a time in the room. Dinner parties in nice bourgeois homes could end in group sex and partner swapping, and pornography was legalized. This was all a result of the sexual revolution. Or was it?

Not really. Even though it felt like moral standards changed radically and the freedom to talk openly about and sexual experimentation emerged over a period of a few years, it was in fact just the culmination of a process that had been going on for many decades. Industrialization of the West had brought material progress, and as living conditions improved people found they had energy for other things besides survival. Women joined the labor force and were suddenly no longer dependent on having to yield to a man for financial security for themselves and their children. If your marriage was unhappy, you could get a divorce.

At the same time, religion lost influence, and living up to Christian norms for sexual behavior became less important. Freud's ideas about the subconscious and the influence of sexuality on human development and behavior had been discussed for over 50 years, and Alfred Kinsey had been snooping into American bedrooms, publishing reports on what he found. In Sweden, Elise Ottosen-Jensen, a journalist and socialist, had fought since the 1920s for a woman's right to have control over her own body and to have access to sexual education, contraception and abortion. In Denmark, the author Agnes Henningsen, mother of the designer Poul Henningsen, had openly lived out her ideals on a woman's right to a self-chosen and varied erotic life since the turn of the century. She suffered strong condemnation from a society that wasn't remotely ready for this.

And in the early sixties, the pill came on the market. Suddenly there was easily accessible and safe contraception that could be administered by the women themselves. The fear of an unwanted pregnancy no longer stopped men and women from going to bed together when desire overwhelmed them. For those who were unlucky and got pregnant anyway, abortion in the first months of pregnancy was legalized in the seventies, and the back-alley abortion clinics, which put women's lives at risk, were history.

So this entire historical process may in fact be the reason for the considerable change in the attitudes toward sex of 70-year-old Swedes from 1976 to 2000. The people interviewed in 1976 were 30 years old in 1936 and in the middle of adulthood when providing information on contraception was still not permitted and homosexuality was forbidden by law for an additional eight years. The people interviewed in 2000 were 30 years old in 1960 - this was the beginning of the welfare boom, just before the contraceptive pill became generally accessible, when women left their kitchen stoves for a pay check and the sexual revolution really took off.

Now television is showing so-called reality shows, where sex is the most important part of the concept, and where all participants – young men and women alike – are sexually assertive and determined to have their desires satisfied. Generally, sex is a big thing in the media, and if it's possible to spice a story up a bit and make it sell better by throwing in some sex, then that's what's done.

However, openness and acceptance are two different things. In 2011, a survey of Danish primary school teachers found that their students still considered a girl who showed too much interest in sex to be cheap.

The Influence of Religion

Although views of sexuality in our part of the world have become more accepting in recent decades, there is still something decadent about sexual desire. It triggers associations with dimly lit rooms, heavy curtains, black lace and perfume. But no one would ever have had the idea to engage in a sexual act if it weren't for the pleasure and satisfaction that comes with it. We are talking about strong forces here, something all cultures have had to realize and take into account.

There has always been a need for societies to control the sexuality of its citizens, to establish rules and laws ensuring that people don't have sex when and with whomever they please. Social order would not last long if they did. Honorable members of the society would resort to murder and fraud, putting fortunes, marriages and personal reputations at risk, and chaos would ensure. Stable, well-functioning families are a necessary basis for a well-functioning society. It doesn't necessarily have to be based on the classic nuclear family with mom, dad and 2.1 kids - it may just as well be large family groups, clans or tribes, as long as there is some kind of order keeping people at bay. Lust and desire must only be allowed in steady relationships where children can safely be born and provided for.

Within marriage, there are rarely any restrictions for sexual activity, at least for men. Sex before marriage may also be acceptable for men, as long as the other participant is not a married woman. Sex outside marriage is normally not acceptable, but often tolerated - again primarily for men. Society, and sometimes also the law, tends to subject women to other rules. Women need to be watched over, and that's how it has been throughout the ages in societies where men are the dominant and powerful sex. Women are never in doubt that their children are really theirs, but men can never be one hundred percent sure. So when men use their power to keep their spouses in tight reins, it is basically an effort to ensure that they are not supporting other men's offspring.

When the aim is to keep the erotic activities citizens in check, religion is often responsible for the rules dictating when, how and with whom sex is permitted to take place. As mentioned, sex is a powerful force, and when sex is in your thoughts, it is difficult to achieve peace of mind and concentrate on the prayers and meditation that bring you closer to God. If you want to achieve high spirituality, the recommended method is to refrain completely from all types of sexual activity.

Religions often group people into different categories: Those who are truly superior, holy or possibly saint-like, living in complete chastity. Then there are the average people who live in well-organized frameworks and families, have sex and raise the children needed to maintain a society. Finally, we have the riffraff, who are unable to control their urges and desires, those who provide sex for money and those who have "illegitimate" children.

But there are differences in how the major religions relate to sex and eroticism, and Christianity seems to be characterized by being the least sex-friendly of them all. For example, the Catholic Church and several fundamentalist Protestant schools of thought still prohibit all types of contraception in an attempt to ensure that sex is only a means of procreation, and not something people do for love, pleasure, and fun. Both Christianity and Buddhism acknowledge, albeit a little reluctantly, that sex is necessary to produce new generations, but the ideal way of life is a spiritual one, focusing on the soul and not the body, and avoiding sex altogether. This can be achieved by living as a monk or a nun, completely separated from the other sex, so you are not tempted and led into depravity by following carnal desires.

The Apostle Paul, author of the oldest texts in the New Testament, clearly expressed that if possible, everybody should live in celibacy like he did himself, completely abstaining from sex and marriage. Marriage should only be entered into if it couldn't be avoided; marriage is only for people who are unable to control their sexual desires. As far as we know, Jesus never married, and there are no indications that he was ever involved in any kind of erotic activities or had any desire to be. Buddha had a wife and child, as long as he was Prince Siddhartha, but left them when he became Buddha. From that moment, he lived in sexual abstinence.

Mohammed however, had several wives and a hoard of children and apparently was sexually active most of his adult life. Islam has traditionally a somewhat more positive attitude toward sex and eroticism than both Christianity and Buddhism, as long as it takes place between husband and wife.

One example is the book *The Perfumed Garden*, written by Sheikh Nefzaoui in the 16th century. It is full of sensual stories of passionate men and women taking pleasure in seducing and satisfying each other in different ways. Lust and desire is permitted and promoted as fully for women as for men, and eroticism and sex are means of pleasure and delight to be engaged in for their own sake. Sex is a way of expressing love. Sex and eroticism are necessary to keep a marriage alive and well, and both spouses are in fact obliged to provide sexual pleasure to their partner.

But a positive attitude toward erotic pleasure is not the same as accepting sexual freedom. There is no such thing in Islam or in any of the other major religions, especially not for women.

Madonnas and Whores

In almost every culture, the rules applying to women's sexual exploits are much stricter than those for men. For women, the prohibition of sex outside of marriage is absolute and definitely not to be trifled with. A chaste Christian woman has traditionally been synonymous with a woman who does not show any interest in sex. She does not take any sexual initiative, and she has sex only because it is a duty to satisfy her husband and to obtain the necessary pregnancies. Just think of how the Catholic church worships the Virgin Mary, a woman who was so chaste and so virtuous that she managed to be impregnated without ever having slept with a man - and how that same church to this day still condemns not only sex before marriage and abortion, but also contraception. Sex is *not* for fun.

This lack of sexual freedom goes hand in hand with restrictions in other areas of social and political life. It is no coincidence that women in Scandinavia, who have a high degree of sexual freedom, were also among the first in the world to be granted the right to vote, regardless of income and marital status. Women have a value as individuals, not only as an appendage to a man - father, husband, brother or son. In much of the world, the woman's role is still to submit to men, to take care of the home and family, and if she doesn't want to do this, she has few opportunities to achieve financial support or even earn a living.

In parts of India, women are of so little value that they can be raped and the perpetrator can go unpunished. Female fetuses and newborn baby girls are killed; widows are burned or relegated to live as beggars. In Saudi Arabia, it is still forbidden for women to be alone with men they are not related to, to go out without a male relative and to drive a car. If a woman reports a rape, she will be punished, as this is tantamount to a confession of having participated in fornication. If she is unmarried, she will be punished with 100 lashes. And if she is married, she has been her unfaithful to her husband – an even more serious crime punishable by death by stoning.

In some countries, particularly in Africa, female genital mutilation is still practiced in an attempt to remove women's sexual desire and increase their value on the marriage market. The Turkish-Kurdish-German lawyer and women's rights activist Seyran Ates has shared with the world how, as a child, she was not allowed to eat popsicles or bananas in the street or other public places, because it could remind bystanders of oral sex, and of course nice girls must never be associated with any kind of sexual act.

So in the eyes of religion, desire is bad, and desire in women even worse. To have sexual desire is a sin, something to be ashamed of. And as we all know, Eve was the one who brought both sin and shame into the world by accepting the fruit offered to her by the snake from the tree of knowledge. The snake was, according to the legends, the woman Lilith, who was Adam's first wife. Unlike Eve, she was not created from Adam's rib, but from the earth like Adam himself and therefore his equal. Lilith left Adam because she would not submit to him. Taught by experience, God created a somewhat tamer female version from Adam's rib.

This old legend, much older than the Bible, has been the excuse for oppression of women, misogyny and direct hatred of women throughout history. The Fall of Man was proof of woman's weak character and inferior morals. It has been used to justify keeping women completely out of the hierarchy and power structures of the church and consequently in society in general. Even today, Christian fundamentalists oppose women becoming priests.

A special chapter in the history of religion is the period 1400–1700, when the witch trials swept through Europe. The witchcraft courts accused mainly women and particularly women over 50. The accused were often strong, competent women who lived alone, were self-sufficient and were often considered forces to be reckoned with. The women identified as witches were accused of putting the evil eye on the neighbor's cow, so it stopped producing milk, they were blamed for diseases and crop failures, but a great many of the allegations against them were explicitly sexual in nature. They caused men to become impotent, and above all, they had wild and shameless sex with the devil himself.

In 1484, the extremely superstitious Pope Innocentius VIII issued a papal declaration stating that there could be no doubt that witches really existed. And to have any other opinion was considered heresy. He subsequently ordered the two Dominican monks, Heinrich Kramer and Jacob Sprenger, to write a complete guide on how to recognize witches, and how they should be handled once captured. The two monks produced the three-volume manual *Malleus Malificarum* (The Hammer of Witches), which includes a titillating collection of kinky sexual fantasies, conceived by the two sex-renouncing gentlemen. The following discussion about the devil and whether it was possible to spot him as he was having a hot encounter with a witch is a prime example:

> "As to whether they commit these abominations together visibly or invisibly, it is to be said that, in all the cases of which we have had knowledge, the devil has always operated in a form visible to the witch; for there is no need for him to approach her invisibly, because of the pact of federation with him that has been expressed. But with regard to any bystanders, the witches themselves have often been seen lying

on their backs in the fields or the woods, naked up to the very navel, and it has been apparent from the disposition of those limbs and members which pertain to the venereal act and orgasm, as also from the agitation of their legs and thighs, that, all invisibly to the bystanders, they have been copulating with Incubus devils; yet sometimes, howbeit this is rare, at the end of the act a very black vapour, of about the stature of a man, rises up into the air from the witch."

Translation from Latin by Rev. Montague Summers, 1928)

This was no doubt dirty, lustful sex, and the description was intended to arouse disgust and condemnation. It worked. In Denmark, about 1,000 people were burned as witches, mostly during the reign of King Christian IV who was himself an active and committed participant in the Danish witch trials.

Countries and Customs

The Australian anthropologist Katrina Moore is one of several researchers to be intrigued by the low sexual activity of older Japanese people. In an effort to find the cause, she interviewed elderly Japanese people of both sexes, and the results are published in a report from 2010. The women describe, somewhat embarrassed, how they have not been permitted to express sexual or erotic desire, not even in marriage. In the early years of marriage, a woman might take the initiative to have sex, but this desire must be expressed in code. For instance, she might serve a special type of seafood for dinner or arrange a small pillow in a special way on the common futon before bedtime. Their husbands, however, had completely different conditions. It was not uncommon for them to have mistresses, even in the early years of marriage, a fact that further contributed to the women withdrawing from the sexual relationship.

When so many restrictions are placed on sexual desire and all its expressions, it is unsurprising that many of the women, already at a young age, stop being sexually active, and that only one out of eight Japanese women over 40 consider sex an important part of life.

But the situation in Japan is not unique. Things are apparently just as bleak in Japan's giant neighbor, China. There it is clear that sexual desire has had a rough time for centuries and it still does. According to a fairly recent study of older people's sexual activity in China, over a third of elderly Chinese people believe it is simply unnatural for older people to have sex. Almost as many think it is downright harmful.

The Chinese mindset is characterized by Confucianism, which is more a philosophy than a religion. In Confucianism, there are strict rules for how the individual must behave to be part of the family, society and the political system. In order to maintain harmony, it is crucial that everyone knows their place in the hierarchy and submits to this system. Minion to prince, wife to husband, children to parents and so on. In traditional Chinese society the woman's role was to take care of the home and to give birth to sons. As a child she was expected to obey her father, when married her husband, as a widow her sons. Daughters were insignificant; they only stayed in the family temporarily and were married off at a young age. Sex was a duty that had to be met in order for families to have sons, and desire or pleasure clearly was not important.

In many ways it is still taboo in China to talk about sex, about sexual problems and techniques, about what good sex is and how to achieve it. Foreplay, oral sex and sex toys are completely unfamiliar concepts for many people in China.

Chinese men may still expect women to simply throw themselves on the back whenever a man wants sex. A research team in the United States set out to examine attitudes about rape among men from East Asian countries and the United States, respectively. Nearly 400 male university students were presented with a story where a woman invites a man she already knows into her home. They have a drink and chitchat. The story ends with the man raping the woman.

The students were asked to indicate whether they thought the incident could be defined as rape, who was to blame for what happened, and whether the woman was really credible when she tried to get the man to stop what he was doing. And there was a difference. The Asian men were more likely than the Americans to believe that it was not a case of rape, and also that the woman herself was to blame for what happened.

So opinions about sex, the roles of men and women and what constitutes proper behavior differ between Asian and Western men. This also applies to women, only the differences also include the level of sexual desire they feel (or admit to feeling). A group of researchers compared the sexual desire of female young university students in Canada. The women came from two different cultures -

East Asian (primarily Chinese) and Western. The study showed that women from the Western culture had the strongest sex drives. The researchers also found a clear relationship between shame and lack of libido. To examine the extent to which women associated sex with shame, participants were asked to what extent they agreed to statements such as: "When I have sex, I enjoy it like all healthy people" or "If I feel sexual desire, I fight against it, because I must have full control over my body". The more the women felt ashamed about wanting to have sex, the lower they rated their desire.

But as the change in the two groups of 70-year-old Swedes shows us, values can change. If you are moved from one culture to another, your opinion about how things should be often also changes, although this does not happen from one day to the next. Many researchers have found differences between Western and East Asian groups with regard to sexual behavior and views on sexual issues. But research also shows that when Asians move to the West and integrate into the new culture, their views on sexuality also change, and sex becomes a greater source of joy rather than something to be ashamed about.

Shame is a very potent means when people have gone astray from the rules of society and need to be knocked back into place. If the desire for sex and eroticism is labeled shameful, desire gradually shrinks away. A Tamil woman wrote in a magazine:

> "I am 56 years old. My husband is almost 70. We live with our son and daughter-in-law.
>
> My husband is still interested in having sex with me, even though I'm not the least interested. We argue a lot because of

this. When I give in to his demands and sleep with him in private at night, I cannot look my daughter in law in the eyes in the morning. I'm dying of shame. I want a solution to this problem. How can I change my husband's attitude and make him understand that what he is doing is wrong?"

This woman clearly lives in a culture where having sex after the woman's childbearing years have passed is not acceptable. And her housing situation, living with her son and daughter-in-law, does not make it any easier.

In the Western world most children move away from home when they are grown up, and for good and bad, it is not very common for several generations to live under the same roof. But elsewhere in the world things are different, and elderly parents often move in to live with one of their married sons. In these cases, the elderly may be required to share a room with their grandchildren or sleep in the sitting room. And why should they need privacy, when it's assumed that at their age, sex is a closed chapter?

A prerequisite for following and enjoying your sexual desire is the possibility to be undisturbed (unless showing off turns you on). Not many people wish to flaunt their sex lives. You don't want to make love spontaneously in your sunny living room on a Saturday afternoon, if there is a risk that your 17-year-old son will suddenly appear on the doorstep with a couple of friends. Teenagers or adult children still living at home can be a significant obstacle to your frolicking in the double bed and elsewhere. They go to bed late, suddenly they may be in the bathroom right next to you or passing the bedroom door, so you are always on guard, ready to muffle your sounds or abstain from sex altogether just in case.

Not all cultures have associated sex with shame and modesty. In Hawaii, life followed some rather different rules until Captain Cook landed in 1778. Sex was considered a source of joy, fun and pleasure for everyone. Modesty was unknown and the climate fantastic, so it was not necessary to wear any clothes. Children were prepared for the joy of sex and encouraged to be sexually active as they reached puberty.

Sex took place openly, and age was apparently no limit. It was not a society completely without rules for dating, but the rules applied mainly to the women, who as a tribal chief ranked highest on the social ladder. They were not permitted to have sex with men of a lower social class. They were also the only ones for whom being a virgin was assigned a value, and that was only the case until they had found a steady partner, one who should also be a tribal chief. From then on it was perfectly acceptable to have lovers on the side, and the children who were born as a result of the relationships were brought up in extended families, based on the lineage of the mother. The inheritance laws - dealing more with social status than material goods - also followed the female line.

The Christian missionaries who arrived in Hawaii 40 years after Cook must have been shaken to their very depths by this pagan disorder. They saw to it that things were rapidly rectified.

Proper Conduct for Elderly People

You can categorize a person in many different ways. Gender is one of them. At birth you will be defined as either a boy or a girl, and from then on, you will be expected to behave in a way appropriate for either a boy or a girl, defined by the culture you live in. You will be told, in subtle or explicit ways, how to dress, what games to play and what kind of career to choose. If you're a boy, your Christmas present may be guns, cars and a football, while your little sister will have dolls, dresses and beads.

Age is another way to categorize people. Some do it more than others. A Dane reading a Norwegian newspaper may wonder why every person mentioned must have their age stated in brackets after their names, as if this is crucial for the reader to get full value from the news, article etc. But to lump everyone of a certain age together and think that they are alike is unreasonable to say the least. We are not all alike when we are born, and as the years pass and we live our lives, the differences become more and more pronounced.

When you've lived long enough to be categorized as "Older", I suggest that the first thing you should do is look around and note the enormous variation between the individuals in the group of people you now belong to. Some are worn out, tired and sick and may be rapidly approaching life's end, while others are healthy, happy and optimistic, full of plans and initiatives. It will become clear that this great diversity is not really important in the eyes of the world, which generally associates growing older with various kinds of loss.

Aging is a change that is not seen as growth, but as a phasing out. Aging is associated with illness, dependency, ugliness and decay. Youth is associated with beauty, full speed ahead, innovation and productivity. These are all positive words in our culture where young people take center stage in most contexts, and even the middle-aged may be forced upstage. How many TV presenters are over 50? How many people over 50 are actually on TV programs compared to the percentage of the population that is over 50? How many movie roles are played with older actors? And when business cut back, who is made redundant first?

The British sociologist Margaret Simey wrote at the age of 96:

"My eyes were opened when kind but misguided well-wishers organized a surprise birthday party for me when I turned 90. Until then, I had been as active as any of them, deeply involved in volunteer work, committee meetings and consultations. Suddenly, it occurred to them, as it did to me, that I was old.

The transformation was stunning. I was no longer one of them. I was an outsider. I seemed to be in a foreign country. I didn't speak the language. I didn't know the rules. I was no longer me, Margaret, very defiantly my own person. Now I was simply one of a mass of clones, a stereotype, a number, not an individual. I was old and that was all that needed to be said."

Being older now is not the same as it was 100 years ago. Society was rougher then, times were often hard and there was no room for people who weren't able to work. They were marginalized and literally powerless. The well-known techniques of the rule came into use. The old and redundant were ridiculed, made invisible, talked down to and disempowered and made to suffer shame as a burden to society. Disease and hard labor wore people out early, pension rights were non-existent and generally people did not look forward to 20 or more active and independent years after working life was over. If you survived your working age at all and didn't have a family to care for you, you were forced to live in the poorhouse.

Life as an older person could be a good life with you as grandmother sitting in the warm corner by the fireplace, petting the cat and telling stories to your grandkids. But you could just as well be stowed away in a cold spare room left to lie with withering muscles and stinking sores and only the fleas in your mattress for company. Fortunately, this is difficult to imagine today in our part of the world, but when I was a kid in the 1950s, it could still happen.

In 1900, the life expectancy for Danish men was about 50 years of age and for women 55. Now it is 77 and 82, respectively. We are healthier and live longer. But being old is still not popular. Those who don't work don't count as full members of society, but are rather considered a financial burden on the community.

In this context old age is not something to look forward to. On the contrary, most people try to avoid it as long as possible. We have learned that it is important to stay active, to avoid stagnation, to use it or lose it, both muscles and brain mass. And, of course, chronic illness is never something that improves quality of life. We feel better and have more disease-free years if we take care of ourselves, stay fit and keep a positive view of our own old age as a good time in life instead of an era of decline and decay. But keeping fit and healthy has gradually become almost a duty so as not to burden the health care system, the public coffers and aesthetics in public spaces.

It sometimes seems like one of the requirements we need to meet in order to prove that we are youthful and healthy is that we still have an active sex life. But I think it's important to emphasize that we also have a choice here. We shouldn't feel ashamed about growing old, and age-related changes do not necessarily show a lack of dedication to caring for ourselves. We don't have to have the sex life of a 25-year-old at the age of 75 to prove that we have managed to grow old in the "right" way. Perhaps it doesn't matter whether we are still able to do as much as possible of what we did when we were younger. We deserve to fall asleep at night with a clear conscience, without absolutely having crossed fitness, red wine, dietary fiber and sex off our to-do list.

Aging can be considered either a process of decline and decay or a progression towards a new way of experiencing and living in the world. In the first instance, you will regret the fact that sex is not what it once was. In the second, you will welcome the change and the new opportunities for closeness and love that come with growing older.

Why all this focus on religion and culture? Well, because they merge into each other and determine our values and opinions about sexuality and gender, aging, relations between men and women and pretty much everything else. And they are not constants; we change them and they change us. But with the great personal freedom we have achieved in our part of the world, it is up to the individual to weigh their own needs against the surrounding culture's norms and strike a balance that gives them the greatest happiness – also when it comes to their sex lives.

Nahid, Age 55

Shortly after we had arrived in Denmark, some neighbors visited us, and suddenly they asked: "So, what about your sex life? What's it like?" My husband and I looked at each other, and my husband began to tell them, but I became angry and went into the kitchen, and my husband came out to me, and I said, "Why are they asking about these things? It's private! I don't even talk to my sisters about it!" My husband said: "It's normal, they are adults and so are we!" But I said, "No, I won't accept it! If they start talking about it again, then they must leave."

And even now, after having lived in Denmark for many years, talking about these things makes me feel shy. But I have also become a little used to it. For example, if I go swimming, I can manage to change clothes even if there are boys in the locker room. So it's baby steps in the beginning. But I'm still shy; I can't really talk to my husband about these things. And I think that our upbringing failed, because it is necessary to talk about these things, about your needs.

But I also think that when it comes to me – it's too late. My upbringing was finished a long time ago, and now it's all inside my head, how I should behave and talk and with whom. If I'm with my husband, and he asks me what I want, I can tell him, but otherwise not. And this creates some misunderstandings from time to time.
But I've changed. When we came to Denmark, my husband liked to sleep with me every night, and I didn't want to. I was so tired - I had

a thousand other things to worry about, education, if we would be allowed to stay here, the children's problems, this and that.

Men, they are generally good about forgetting everything when they get into bed - we aren't. But I think I'm getting better at helping him to understand that I am not a female rabbit, I can't just go to bed with him ... It should be maybe once a week, when we sit down and talk, maybe have a glass of wine - and then, afterwards. But not that every time he wants to, I'm expected to say yes.

In the beginning he had a very hard time understanding this. He didn't want to accept it, no, when you feel the desire, you should obey it. But if you "must", then it becomes a duty, and not like you go to bed to make love, in the way that your thoughts are with him.

Now we sleep together once, twice, three times a month, and it's okay. He's a little dissatisfied. He says, we have to ... But I say no, we don't have to. You can sleep in that bed and I'll sleep here. When I think of my father-in-law, it was the same - he wanted to, but his wife didn't. She said: "No, we're old people! We should be ashamed!" But he said, "No, we are a married couple, we are living people, so we should also have sex."

I am a Muslim in the sense that I was taught not to lie and to try to help others as much as I can. You don't have to wear veils to show that you are a good Muslim. But according to religious rules ... my husband says that if a man wants to have sex, and the woman says no, she goes straight to hell. I say, well okay, I'd rather go to hell! He says it in a way that makes fun of it, but many Muslim women say that it says in the Qu'ran that you must satisfy your husband. But it depends on what culture you come from. If you come from a very religious family, you do as it's written in the Qu'ran.

We did not have sexual education in school, we don't know anything about these things, and suddenly you are married and nobody has told you anything. I have heard that today the girls in Iran are given some education before getting married. The government ensures this, and I think that young people today know a lot more than we did. I've been too shy to talk to my own girls about these things, but I knew that they heard about them in school and I think it's good that Danish schools teach this.

But generally it's believed in Iran that when you grow old, the sex should end. And old is 50. I know many women who don't remarry if they lose their husband. They think it's shameful. They may have children and in-laws, and it is shameful if they re-marry. The man often marries again if he loses his wife, but women don't, even if it says in the Qu'ran that it is okay to get married again, if you are widowed. They think about the neighbors, friends, family - what would they say if they remarried?

We don't accept adultery in Iran. But I have heard that many men marry a woman that they don't live with, but just visit once in a while. They defend themselves by saying that they can afford it, so why shouldn't they take care of one more woman? And I think it's very wrong, because if a woman is with another man than her husband, she will be convicted and stoned, but the man can just say that he wanted to help another woman financially. I think it's so unfair. But this won't change. As long as there is Iran is an Islamic republic, it will only get worse. Even when they get divorced, the man gets the right to keep the children. And this is why many women accept all these stupid things their husbands do and stay with them because they can't get custody of the children.

If my husband became impotent and we couldn't be together anymore, it would be fine with me, because I don't want to. If my husband didn't ask me for sex for a month or two, it wouldn't hurt me. It wouldn't make any difference to our relationship. I ask him often how long he intends to go on. He wants to continue.

When I lost the desire, he became suspicious and thought that maybe I had another man. But then we went to a psychologist in Iran, who told him that when women are my age, there are other things that concern them: their career and work, and their families. Sexual life is at the bottom of the list. And the man may have to spend all week making his woman ready, there is no use thinking that you can have a fight, and an hour later the man can have sex. We're not animals - we are humans, we have feelings. I had more desire when I was younger, but ... I can't remember when I had my last orgasm.

Body, Aging, Hormones, and Sex

Even if we want to, we can't ignore the fact that as we grow older our bodies can't perform as they did when we were younger. Our senses grow a bit duller. Our muscles slowly become weaker until one day we find ourselves wonder how a young person can lift a heavy box or pull a stubborn cork out of a wine bottle with so little effort. Flexibility and balance decrease, and you find that it's safest to sit on the edge of the bed while putting on your socks so you don't topple over. For a while, we take your glasses off and on constantly until we surrender to the inevitable bifocals.

Our skin also changes. It grows thinner, less elastic and looser in structure. It is more easily bruised and heals more slowly. Gravity starts to gain power over forms - breasts, buttocks and stomach are slowly pulled downward. Cheeks settle down around the chin, which may in turn slip a little down the neck. Facial features start to show all the joys and sorrows we have encountered in life. And where young people have bodies that clearly illustrate the physical differences between men and women, older people tend to look more alike. It is as if the differences in appearance are only necessary as long as we are fertile and prepared to have children, and thus need to be able to signal to each other that we are capable of procreation.

There is not much we can do to influence these changes. They come to all of us if we live long enough. It's all part of the natural aging process. But when it comes down to it, most of us actually have a rather opportunistic attitude toward nature. We usually only agree with nature when it shows it's pretty and pleasant side. Squirrels and songbirds are okay for most; typhoons and rooks are not okay and must be fought. And natural aging is not something that is actually celebrated. Once you've got your driver's license and voting rights, birthday speeches tend to focus on sharp corners in life and time passing too fast.

When it's not possible to overlook the external changes anymore, a whole industry is ready to help us to hide and smooth out the changes. There are dietary supplements that boost memory, smooth the skin, lubricate the joints, increase desire, sharpen vision, eliminate hot flashes and prevent enlarged prostates. There is cosmetic surgery that slims here and fills there. There are creams and ointments that prevent wrinkles and cosmetics to hide those that relentlessly come anyway. There are workout programs that tighten and lift and products that make teeth whiter and hair darker. There are artificial joints, so 80 year olds can play tennis and run marathons, and there is Viagra so men can get erections and have sex like 25 year olds.

When our bodies change, it has to do partly with changes in the levels of various hormones in the blood.

Hormones are the body's messengers. They are substances produced in cells and glands, released into the blood and passed through the body to their target organ, where they act and take effect. They are involved in every single process that makes us living beings. They influence each other in different ways in a complex system and ensure that the body adapts and reacts appropriately in the many situations humans might encounter - hunger, danger, pregnancy and stress, just to mention a few.

Hormones are also affected by the sensory input we constantly receive, conveying what happens around us. What we see and feel, sounds, smells that reach us, all inform us about where we are, whether we are in danger or if it's okay to relax and lower our guard.

If you are crossing a street and suddenly see a car coming toward you, the danger of being run down causes your adrenal glands to secrete adrenaline. Adrenaline causes the heart to beat faster and increases your breathing so that more oxygen reaches your muscles, enabling them to work. You become aware of the approaching danger and the adrenaline has made sure that you are physically able to run safely over on the other side of the road. When you eat and the food reaches your stomach and duodenum, a lot of different hormones are secreted. They affect both how the intestines move and how food is digested and absorbed from the intestines to the blood, as well as whether the nutrients are to be stored in the muscles, liver or fat tissue under the skin or around the intestines.

We wouldn't be able to survive without hormones, but some are more important than others. They are a necessary part of our system to make our bodies grow, develop and function and to enable us to survive as individuals. The sex hormones estrogen and testosterone are special in this regard. They allow humans to survive as a species, but individuals could easily live without them. But they are crucial when it comes to the biological conditions that define us as sexual beings, as men and women. When it comes to our relationships to others and to sex, a lot of other hormones also come into play.

Estrogen

The female hormone estrogen comes predominantly from the ovaries where production begins from the start of puberty as the eggs develop and grow. The effect of estrogen is to make the female body ready for sex and pregnancy. As the amount of estrogen in the blood increases, the body changes, the breasts, hips and buttocks develop.

The lining of the vagina becomes thick and furrowed and covered with lactic acid bacteria providing an acid environment which acts a microbiological barrier. This prevents other microorganisms, like bacteria and Candida, from taking hold and causing inflammation. The vaginal lining also produces a secretion that lubricates and cleans the vagina and creates a hospitable environment for sperm. The mucosa in the uterus grows and becomes ready to accept and nourish a fertilized egg that can develop into a new person. Estrogen also affects the skin and hair. The skin contains more moisture and is more elastic as long as there is estrogen in the blood. The hair is thicker and shinier.

For most women, menopause sets in around the age of 50. This is the period in a woman's life where there are no more eggs in her ovaries and no more estrogen is produced. In the years leading up to menopause, the estrogen levels in the blood may rise and fall steeply within few days. This can be experienced as a tendency to fluctuate in weight and as mood swings, and if the woman is suffering from migraine she may have more attacks. Other symptoms are hot flashes and irregular periods.

When there finally are no more eggs in the ovaries and no more cells which can form estrogen, the body's estrogen level falls relatively abruptly. Then a woman's period stops altogether and pregnancy is no longer possible. For some women this is the only way they register their menopause. Others are not so lucky and can be plagued by hot flashes and sweating for many years.

Eventually there will be physical changes, most clearly felt in places where estrogen has the greatest effect. For instance, it may affect all the mucous membranes, and some women notice a tendency toward dry eyes, which can make it difficult to use contact lenses.

But for most women, the vaginal changes will be the most obvious. Lactic acid bacteria can't thrive where there is no estrogen, and when they disappear, the vagina loses part of its protection against infections. Regardless of how often and with what you wash yourself, there will always be plenty of intestinal bacteria in the genital area. When the lactic acid bacteria disappear and the vagina becomes more vulnerable, the intestinal bacteria are more likely to do harm and, for example, cause vaginal inflammation and discharge. Some women are also more prone to bladder infections.

The mucous membranes of the labia and vagina also become thinner and less elastic, so sex may be a dry and painful affair. If you shave your pubic hair, you may more easily develop a skin infection in the area. But there are also positive effects of lack of estrogen: postmenopausal women rarely develop vaginal yeast infections as the fungus can't thrive where there is no estrogen.

When the production of estrogen stops, the physical changes are obvious. But what about the libido, the desire to have sex? Well, the influence of estrogen on a woman's desire for and enjoyment of sex is much debated. On the one hand, estrogen increases blood flow to the vagina, clitoris and labia, and this could make it easier for women to become sexually aroused.

On the other hand, there is nothing to suggest that women have more sex when they are given estrogen supplements. If a woman suffers from declining interest in sex after menopause, it does not help to give her an estrogen supplement unless the lack of desire is caused by the simple fact that it hurts to have sex because the vagina has become dry and vulnerable. So while estrogen is essential for a woman's fertility, is does not seem to have much influence on her desire.

Testosterone

Just as girls' ovaries begin producing estrogen at the start of puberty, boys' testicles produce testosterone, the primary male sex hormone. This hormone is not only crucial when it comes to men's sexual function, it is also important for women as it stimulates desire and makes the body ready for sex. It increases the libido in both sexes, and the more testosterone people have in their blood, the more often their thoughts are preoccupied with sex (and yes, most people do actually think about sex several times each day).

While men, and also women after menopause, have testosterone levels that are fairly stable from day to day, ovulating women have testosterone levels that change throughout the month and peak just before ovulation. If a woman's sex life was entirely controlled by her own desire, she would go looking for a sexual partner at exactly this time, which is also the time of her cycle when sex may result in a pregnancy. When a woman is taking contraceptive pills, these spikes in her testosterone levels are leveled out, and women sometimes register this as a loss of, especially, the mid-cycle libido. This can be so annoying that some women choose to stop taking the pills altogether.

Testosterone is also a real macho hormone. But macho men are not only sexy, they also live dangerous lives. High levels of testosterone make people of both sexes prone to taking risks, and while risk taking can be good and lead to fast action when necessary, to progress and development, it can also make people overly confident and reckless, like when very young, testosterone-pumped men feel immortal and end up killing themselves at 100 mph. People's willingness to take risks shows in their choice of career, their hobbies, the way they invest their money and probably also the kinds of movies they like and what books they read.

It is well-known fact in the medical world that a doctor's choice of specialization matches their personality: pediatricians are kind;

psychiatrists sensitive, endocrinologists are nerdy and like to wear ties... Some years ago, a Danish newspaper asked nurses which medical specialization had the sexiest male doctors. The winners were anesthesiologists and orthopedic surgeons, both specializations with a lot of drama and action, and they were the clear preference if the nurses wanted to party and have a great night out. But if they wanted someone to marry, they tended to go for a pediatrician or a GP (which says as much about the nurses as the doctors). Pathologists and psychiatrists were considered boring. If doctor's testosterone levels were checked, it would certainly show significant differences between the various medical specializations.

Both men and women react with a prompt increase in testosterone when they become aware of somebody attractive nearby. So testosterone is important in stimulating desire, but it also has other very important effects. It is very important for a person's general vigor. Low testosterone levels, at least if you're a man, could mean your life expectancy may be shorter than average. Some might argue that this wouldn't really matter, seeing as how it would probably be a pretty boring life anyway.

As mentioned before, men with low testosterone levels are less prone than others to taking risks, and maybe this is why they are also less attractive to the opposite sex. A woman has different ways of assessing a man's testosterone level. First, she can sniff her way to it, and second, she can see it in his facial features. Research shows a correlation between men's testosterone levels and features that women perceive as distinctly masculine. And women want sex with macho-men, at least at the time of month when they are most fertile.

However, in the period after ovulation, when a woman may have become pregnant, her preferences change, and she prefers a man with lower testosterone levels and probably, all things considered, a milder appearance. There may be good sense in this, unless she wants a man who would rather take care of his car than his baby.

Men don't have a well-defined transition where their fertility suddenly disappears and their hormone levels drop. Instead, their age-related changes come gradually over the years. The level of testosterone in a man's blood already begins to decrease in his twenties, and it steadily and relentlessly declines throughout his life. A high level of male hormone makes it easier for muscles to grow, and young men don't have to pump much iron to look very strong.

However, things are different when you're 70. It is still possible to achieve strong and impressive muscles at that age, but you just have to work a lot harder for it, and if you aren't careful about staying fit, you will discover that you lose your muscles fairly quickly. This is one of the reasons why old people quickly become weak if they are confined to a bed.

A declining testosterone level also means a man has to work harder to avoid fat depositing around his waist. His hair growth changes, too: it tends to disappear from his head and lower legs and increase on his back and in his ears. It takes longer to get an erection and maybe also to reach climax, a change that may be welcomed by men with a tendency for premature ejaculation.

For some men, not only does it take longer to get an erection, the penis may not be able to become stiff enough for intercourse and maintaining an erection can also be a problem. It is not uncommon to notice a change already from the age of 40, and when men are over 75, almost half of them indicate that their erections are not what they once were. These changes are not caused by low testosterone, however, but far more often by atherosclerosis, or hardening of the arteries.

Testosterone has an effect on desire, but not so much on the ability to maintain an erection long enough to have satisfying intercourse. So if a man feels a strong enough desire, but still can't get an erection, he should look for another reason besides low testosterone. After an orgasm the older man needs a longer period of restitution than when he was younger, so while a 20-year-old is able to have sex many times a day, once a week or less may be enough for an 80-year-old. And his mind is less likely to be occupied by sexual thoughts than when he was younger.

Testosterone is significant for the overall well-being of women as well, for their muscular strength and their physical ability. If debilitated, elderly women with chronic heart problems are given a testosterone supplement, they perform better. Their muscles become stronger and it also enables them to walk faster and for longer distances. Just as for men, women's testosterone levels decrease steadily throughout adult life, and unlike estrogen, there is not a marked reduction when menopause sets in. So if a woman's sexual desire suddenly disappears after menopause, it is rarely due to hormonal changes.

Can men suffer from too little testosterone? At times, there have been speculations about whether men have a transition similar to women's menopause which could give them symptoms of low testosterone in much the same way as women can experience hot flashes, thin mucous membranes and so on. This would make them potential customers for testosterone supplements, so the question has had considerable attention from the pharmaceutical industry. But as mentioned before, men don't experience the same abrupt changes in sex hormone levels that women do; testosterone levels decrease slowly from the age of 20.

However, even though it happens gradually, some men will at some point have testosterone levels so low that it affects their well-being. And in such cases, treatment can be beneficial. A man should consider having his testosterone level checked if he notices a sudden decrease in libido, if his erections become weaker or disappear completely or if his strength, energy and endurance decrease. In fact, the symptoms of low a testosterone level and depression are quite similar, and low a testosterone level can cause depression and vice versa. But there is one significant difference between the two conditions. A certain sign that a man is suffering from testosterone deficiency and not depression is that he won't have to shave as often as before.

Prolactin

Prolactin, the lactation hormone, has a significant influence on sexuality and procreation. This hormone is very important for parent's attachment to their child, and it was probably what caused a young first-time mother in the maternity ward, completely enamored in her newborn daughter, to declare: "I feel so sorry for all the other mothers who have such ugly babies when mine is so beautiful!"

A high level of prolactin will keep the other sex hormones low. This is very important for children and young animals, because it means that their parents are more attentive to the needs of their minors than to roaming around the surroundings in search of sexual partners.

A good example is the emperor penguin. In this species, the parents divide the family tasks between them in a beautiful and efficient way. After the females have laid the eggs, they go out to sea and feed on fish, leaving the males to sit on the eggs alone. During this period, which lasts several months, the males stand still with the egg between their knees, so the chick can grow inside the egg, despite the Arctic cold, snow and ice. The level of prolactin in the blood of the males increases after mating, and this drives them to put their own needs aside and care for their offspring. When the females return, well-fed and healthy, they take over caring for the newly hatched young, and now is the males' turn to go convalesce at the edge of the ice along with the other new fathers. But the male is still under the influence of high levels of prolactin, so he doesn't forget his family. As soon as he has put on a bit of weight after the tough nesting period, he goes back and the parents work together to feed and care for their chick.

In a pregnant woman, the level of prolactin increases during pregnancy, and it remains elevated as long as she is breastfeeding. The high amount of prolactin in her blood suppresses the sex hormones, and therefore it is not uncommon for breastfeeding women to suffer from vaginal dryness and decreased sex drive.

Fortunately, not only the mother winds down hormonally to concentrate on the baby. A man who has just become a father also has higher levels of prolactin and less testosterone in his body than men without children. And the men who have the highest levels of prolactin and lowest levels of testosterone in their blood are the ones who are most alert to the baby's crying and other signals indicating an urgent need for father or mother.

So prolactin is a real parental care hormone, but it also serves a sex-related function. During intercourse or other sexual activity it increases a little, but immediately after orgasm there is a sharp rise and it takes a couple of hours before it gets back to normal. In this setting, prolactin apparently helps to evoke the feeling of calm and satisfaction that comes after good sex. And this sense of well-being created by prolactin doesn't change as you grow older and haven't had to care for your offspring for many years. Good sex will still be good sex.

Oxytocin

Like prolactin, oxytocin is important for giving birth and caring for the baby. It causes the uterus to contract during labor in order to make the cervix open and then to push the baby gradually through the birth canal and out into the world. During breast feeding it causes the mammary glands to contract and excrete milk through the nipples.

But oxytocin is also an important element in entirely different processes involved in interaction between people. This makes it of interest to areas of research in human behavior. One such area is neuroeconomics, a multidisciplinary field dealing with, among other things, how we make decisions and interact with others to make a certain choices. A choice requires a rapid calculation in the mind, a quick weighing of the pros and cons, and although we aren't always aware of what lies in the scales, the number one question is always: "What's in it for me?"

Oxytocin can affect what we regard as the right outcome of our choice. Take the following experiment, for instance:

In an ingenious collaboration between neuroeconomists and psychologists, one group of men received oxytocin and another group received a placebo. They were then asked to play a game where they were each given 100 dollars. They can choose to give a portion or the entire sum to an opponent, and as bait the transaction itself tripled the amount given. If they chose to give 20 pounds away, the opponent in fact received 60 pounds. The opponent can then choose to say thanks by giving an amount back, but he can also choose not to give anything. The opponent was either a human or a computer. It turned out that the men who were treated with oxytocin gave more than twice as much to the opponent as the ones who had received the placebo. But they did so only if the opponent was a human, because then it was hoped that this man would decide that they should both get something out of it.

The men treated with oxytocin thus had confidence in their opponent making common cause with them. They were also well aware of the fact that there was no reason to expect social behavior or empathy if the opponent were a computer. The men who had received the placebo showed exactly the same amount of skepticism to people and machines.

The conclusion of this experiment was that oxytocin causes us to feel more confidence in other people, but not to take more risks.

Oxytocin is closely related to the sense of well-being that comes from trusting others, being part of a social network and being able to enter into relationships with other people. Oxytocin has also been called a love hormone because it appears to provide peace, trust and satisfaction and a feeling of being more confident and comfortable with your partner. Being caressed, cuddled or having a massage causes oxytocin levels to rise, and when you pet your dog, oxytocin increases as well - both in yourself and in the dog. High oxytocin levels increase our resistance to stress and enable us to recover faster after stressful experiences.

When we have sex, the level of oxytocin increases, and during orgasm we're flooded with it. This applies to both men and women, and oxytocin is just like prolactin: Whether we are 20 years old or 80, sex has this very beneficial effect on our minds and well-being.

We can conclude that it is possible to manipulate people's oxytocin levels and thus potentially fiddle with their emotions and behavior. It therefore comes as no surprise that you can buy oxytocin online, for instance as a spray with the alluring name Liquid Trust. A small amount each morning and evening, and then, according to the advertisement, you will not only meet your one and only, but also become a better salesperson and give your career a turbo boost. In this context, I think it's appropriate to emphasize that your personal appearance and behavior are far more influenced by what you believe there is in the bottle than by what it actually contains. A company with convincing marketing and a product that claims to help people fulfill their innermost wishes could probably make money selling sand in the Sahara.

Dopamine

Dopamine is not a hormone but a so-called neurotransmitter, a substance that mediates signals from one nerve cell to another. There are a myriad of neurotransmitters in the brain, which affect each other and affect different areas of the brain. These are very complex mechanisms, and a great deal of them are not yet identified or fully understood.

Dopamine participates in many of the brain's various functions, and if they are disrupted because of too much or too little dopamine or by a change in sensitivity to dopamine in an area of the brain, this can affect both body and mind. What dopamine does, among other things, is to teach us when there is a reward in sight and to motivate us to do whatever needed to achieve that reward. And it provides us with the good feeling of having achieved exactly what we wanted, the reward.

Here's an example: Picture yourself sitting on your sofa one evening, and suddenly you remember that there's a delicious piece of chocolate in the kitchen cupboard. You can't stop imagining yourself unwrapping it, putting it in your mouth and sensing the full and sweet flavor – you've tasted chocolate before, so you know this.

Finally, you can't resist the temptation and you go to the kitchen and find the chocolate. This is dopamine at work. When you have once learned that something is good, dopamine makes you try to find it again. And afterwards, when your needs have been met, the nerve cells that were active as a result of dopamine can relax for a while. You have no immediate need for more. At least not for the first few minutes. Then you may begin to feel that it really wasn't enough with one piece, and the urge to raid the kitchen cupboard arises again. It works in exactly the same way with sex. When you have had great sex once, you come back for more, again and again.

Without dopamine you would still know that chocolate was in the kitchen, but you would not think of it as a source of pleasure or develop the urge to eat it. You might think now that the perfect life must be completely free of dopamine. No cravings for chocolate or other treats, no unmet needs, total freedom from all desires. But then you would also lose the ability to satisfy your vital and natural needs, such as thirst and hunger, and you would not survive that for very long.

As for sex, you would probably feel desire, while the motivation to move on, find a partner and have sex with her or him would not be there.

In the context of evolution, dopamine is an ancient chemical that is necessary for us as living creatures to eat, reproduce, and quench our thirst. But unfortunately you can become addicted to rewarding yourself, also with harmful things. Drugs, alcohol and nicotine, shopping and gambling, for example, are all things that can cause a rapid and strong sense of having fulfilled a need. Some of these are such strong dopamine activators that already after trying them just once, you're hooked and willing to put everything else aside. Try sex instead - under normal circumstances, it's cheaper and less dangerous.

Desire, Arousal and Satisfaction

In Plato's *The Republic* Socrates asks the aging Cephalus what it's like to be old and whether he misses the pleasures of youth. Cephalus answers that old age as such is not a major problem and continues:

> "How well I remember the aged poet Sophocles, when in answer to the question, How does love suit with age, Sophocles, — are you still the man you were? Peace, he replied; most gladly have I escaped the thing of which you speak; I feel as if I had escaped from a mad and furious master. His words have often occurred to my mind since, and they seem as good to me now as at the time when he uttered them. For certainly old age has a great sense of calm and freedom; when the passions relax their hold, then, as Sophocles says, we are freed from the grasp not of one mad master only, but of many."

Sophocles describes his lack of desire as liberation, as getting rid of a "mad and furious master". Desire, the need to have sex, should not be confused with arousal and does not necessarily imply that one imagines being with a particular partner in a certain way. Desire causes sexual thoughts, associations and fantasies. Desire is also being open and receptive to sexual signals and having a tendency to perceive sexual undertones in situations, pictures and statements. The intensity of desire spans over a spectrum from insatiable desire, occupying your mind completely and making you constantly reach for the nearest possible sex partner, to desire that can only be awakened by strong stimulation or can't be awakened at all. The opposite of desire, aversion, exists too, and may cause feelings of disgust at the mere thought of sex.

With desire comes a need to follow it, to quench your thirst (this is the dopamine again), and the expectation that it will bring satisfaction. Sexual satisfaction is equal to getting your needs filled, no matter how big or small they are. The aging Sophocles was completely satisfied – he didn't have any sex life, and he didn't want any.

Desire is a complex, volatile and vulnerable feeling that is easily affected by most of life's circumstances. It matters how comfortable you are with yourself and your life. If you are ill, stressed, depressed or tired, desire can elude you. If you are insecure about whether you're attractive enough, ashamed of your body, in doubt about whether you're a good enough sex partner, then your negative feelings about yourself make it hard for desire to unfold. Perhaps you also have to negotiate with your own sexual morality to approve of your desire. Do you welcome desire, or is there a stern preacher somewhere in your mind, ready with cold showers and slaps on the wrists if your hands aren't visible on top of the quilt? Do you see yourself as a lovesick old fool, who ought to have forgotten all about sex long ago? Or vice versa: Are you concerned that desire is not there at all?

A partner can have major influence on your desire, both positive and negative. You play up to each other, throw fuel on the fire, cause it to grow, want to be close, to touch and sense each other, give and receive pleasure and love. You define yourselves as a couple and as lovers, as two belonging together: you may have quarreled and want to show that you are friends again. Or perhaps things are at the other end of the scale and your partner doesn't turn you on anymore. You may have sex just to keep the peace at home. Or you may actually be repelled by the idea of intimacy at all levels, and don't involve yourself in sex at all.

Sex is perceived as a natural part of human life. A quick Google search shows that there are far more concerns about too little desire than about too much. Lack of desire is something that creates genuine anxiety, especially among young people. "- Is there something wrong with me? - I love my husband - why don't I want sex as often as he does? - Why does my wife only want to have sex twice a week – I'm desperate, doesn't she love me anymore? "

Besides all the external factors that vary throughout life and affect our sexual drive, there are two important things we cannot run away from. One is gender. Men have consistently higher sex drives than women. Women of all age groups score lower on the desire scale than men of a similar age. In addition, a man's sex drive is apparently less sensitive to external influence than a woman's, whose sexuality in general seems more flexible than a man's. Where men's desires, sexual interests and attitudes are fairly constant throughout life, women seem more changeable, adapting to the situation they are in. Compared to men, women's sexuality seems to a greater extent to be influenced by factors such as education and religiousness, where both low education and a high degree of religiousness make women more reluctant to try different sexual experiences and also less likely to use contraception. Women who move from one culture to another also adapt to the new culture's sexual norms to a greater extent than men.

All cultures demand more adjustment of desire and sexuality from women than from men. Women who are unable to adapt are excluded, like my old schoolmate Gunilla. A woman's biology is also much more fluctuating than a man's, menstruation, ovulation, pregnancy, lactation and menopause all present different hormonal combinations with varying influence on sexuality.

The second factor that influences desire is age. Just like Sophocles, both men and women typically find that the spontaneous desire decreases over time. The older you get, the less you think about sex: While Swedish men under the age of 35 indicate that they think about sex every day, this is only the case for a third of men over 65.

According to a Danish report from 2002 on the sexuality of 60-year-old women, one third experienced desire every week, while a survey from California, where women between the ages of 40 and 99 were asked about their sex lives, showed that one third of the women surveyed rarely felt sexual desire. But the older they were, the less they cared about it. This applied to older men in the study from Sweden, too. The older they were, the more satisfied they were with their sex lives, regardless of the diminishing desire.

Let's go back to the women in California. One third of them rarely or never felt desire for sex. This was particularly true for the oldest women. But that did not mean that they didn't have sex, because they could easily be aroused. Half of the women over 80 stated that they become aroused and wet when they had sex, but desire was not what made them hit the sheets. It was the other things that make people want sex: a desire to be close and intimate with their beloved, the expectation of well-being during sex and the relaxation afterwards.

This shows that desire is not necessary for a satisfying sex life. Even with a lack of desire, you can become sexually aroused, so that the penis becomes rigid or the vagina becomes wet and you reach orgasm. Arousal is a reaction that depends on the proper stimulation of your senses, on what turns you on - touch, smell, naughty words, pictures or a wonderful mix of everything. And not least it depends on you allowing yourself to get turned on.

However, as you grow older, it may take longer to become excited. Young women can grow moist and young men get an erection within 30 seconds, but when you are older it may take ten minutes or more, if it is even possible at all. As mentioned before, many men have trouble with getting their penis as rigid as in their younger years and also with maintaining rigidity long enough to reach orgasm.

An Australian study of men between the ages of 75 and 95 found that half had erectile dysfunction, and almost as many had less desire for sex than before. Nearly 40 percent could no longer ejaculate. Similarly, a proportion of older women feel that the vagina never gets wet enough, no matter how much they are stimulated.

However, erotic pleasure is multifaceted. What do people really like to do, and what do they want to get out of having sex when they grow older? Is it the same as when they were 25? No, apparently not. With age, orgasm becomes less important, and sensuality, intimacy and long-lasting enjoyment take over. Virtually every study shows that although desire decreases, and it can be more difficult to get excited and reach orgasm as people grow older, overall satisfaction with sex increases. In a way, a balance is achieved between what we want and expect and what we are actually getting. Depending on one's temperament, it may be classified as resignation, wisdom, satisfaction with what's possible, or perhaps the clear-sightedness of old age, what we know as gerotranscendence.

Gerotranscendence

The theory of gerotranscendence was developed by the Swedish sociologist Lars Tornstam in the late eighties. The term stands for a certain change in your mindset when you grow old. It is described as a positive change in a person's development that can entail both wisdom and increased life satisfaction.

At the heart of gerotranscendence is the feeling that life has fallen into place and that you yourself are not so important, but rather part of a larger whole. You don't care so much about small problems anymore. You accept the mysteries of life and that it isn't necessary to understand or make sense of everything, and you become less engaged and self-occupied. Your belongings, your doings and your acquaintances are reviewed, considered and sorted, and you drop what's not important to you anymore and only keep the things and friends that really matter to you. You may also achieve a greater sense of connectedness with both generations who preceded you and those following. You no longer need to dissemble or try to be somebody other than yourself. And you are less afraid of disease and death.

Sounds like something to look forward to, right? Research has shown that people over 50 are happier and more satisfied with their lives than younger people are. But this is only the case as long as you don't wish to be somebody else, somebody other than the person you are. Where sex is concerned, gerotranscendence is only possible if you don't think of the wild desire and unlimited sexual capacity of the 20-year-old as the only thing worth having, but are able to rejoice in the notion that everything in life has its time and its own way.

Per, Age 68

I have been married to Karen for 45 years. We started going out in high school. At that time, you had to get married to get an apartment, so we got married. Actually, we weren't that much into each other, but we had a nice time together.

We had a couple of children and the years passed. And then, during a vacation in a Greek village, we fell in love. We had been married for 21 years by then.

Everything gets better and easier as the years pass. You learn to accept things. You know more patterns when you grow older and you've tried more things in life. There's nothing new under the sun and you follow a kind of script for how you react in certain situations.

She has become more and more beautiful. She's stunning! Sexually, we have polarized each other, become more man and more woman along the way, and that has made it even better. Sex has never been of crucial importance to us, but we hug a lot. It's about six weeks now since we last had sex.

When we do have sex, it's always in the morning on Saturday or Sunday. We often start by giving each other an oil massage. Orgasm is not so important, but the bodily contact is, and pleasure. I'm not able to stay stiff for very long and seldom reach orgasm. She might not either, so sometimes it's a challenge to find out when we're finished, so to speak. I don't really think it would make any difference if I were impotent.

My desire has grown weaker, so the actual sex act is not as important. But our bodies are, touching each other, licking. It's important to us that we're not completely fixated on achieving an orgasm, if we were, one might be ashamed of not managing it. If the purpose was to get the job done, and one couldn't ...

Sex and Disease

Every man desires to live long, but no man wishes to be old, said the writer Jonathan Swift. And the reality of life is that the longer we live, the greater the risk of developing some kind of disease. The risk of serious or chronic illness also increases with time. When our time comes to leave this world, death must have a reason.

Chronic or serious illness changes your self-image. Suddenly you're not the person you once were. You lose control over your life, your freedom of action diminishes, the future becomes unpredictable. The strong and able become weak. The body changes, may look and feel different, does not function the way it used to, has been subjected to procedures, radiation or medication.

It's difficult to feel desirable and attractive, to be a man or a woman for your beloved, when you're tired, in pain, afraid of looking ugly or smelling wrong, and unable to act as you have done in the past. The fear of losing your partner is tangible if you feel you can no longer be the lover you once were and are no longer an erotic inspiration. You may feel that your role in the relationship is altered, that the balance between you and your partner has changed, especially if you become seriously impaired and need help with practical and personal tasks - maybe even as intimate as hygiene and personal care. It can be a challenge for both parties.

However, sex and eroticism can also still provide quality to life in general as well as to the relationship with a partner. This is partly because sex is great and usually makes you feel good, and partly because it is an affirmation of love: The two of us still belong together, even if one of us is sick right now. We still love each other.

If for some reason it is not possible to have sex, there are other ways of finding that sense of belonging together. Most often, it is still possible to be physically close to each other, cuddle a bit and feel the intimacy and confidence. It soothes body and soul, when a harsh, unfair disease and exhausting treatment have got you down.

Cancer

When you are diagnosed with cancer, it is more than just the body's strength and health at stake. It is life itself. It is a sudden and tangible realization that your time in this world really is limited and not infinite. Suddenly you truly understand that you will one day die, not just some time in the future but possibly soon. Your foothold in life, the familiar daily life, disappears altogether. From one day to the next your life changes completely, and it will never be the same.

Regardless of the type of cancer you are diagnosed with, the shock and worry and fear of death will affect your sex drive. There's just no room for sex and passion in your life when you've got a life-threatening illness. But at the same time, physical contact with another human being is incredibly rewarding. Nothing provides comfort and support like being held in somebody's arms when you need it. Amid all the sickness, it is also important to be able to feel that eroticism still exists, that you are still loved and that while there's so much more at stake, your relationship with your partner is still there and unthreatened. And even when things look dark and hopeless, you are allowed to hope for a life after treatment, where there's also a place for desire and sex.

When somebody is diagnosed with cancer, the course of treatment is often described as a fight or a battle and this is not without reason. It is demanding and hard, both physically and mentally. Cancer is a violent and aggressive enemy to be up against, and the weapons to fight it have to be equally powerful. The necessary treatment for destroying the cancer will also have an effect on the rest of the body.

Cancer treatment usually means surgery, radiation therapy or chemotherapy or a combination of all three. The various therapies attack the cancer in different ways, but they all have the side effect that you feel tired and physically run down for a period, and they can all affect both sexual desire and the ability to become aroused and reach orgasm. Operations on or near the genitals can have a direct impact on your sex life by altering genital anatomy and appearance, or by injuring blood vessels and nerves with the consequence that sensation and reflexes do not work as before. Men can have erectile problems, women vaginal dryness.

After an operation you may also have to face the fact that your body has been changed forever. There may be a scar or a colostomy or a breast has been removed. You may experience a new shyness, an urge to hide your body, even from a partner with whom you have shared most of your life. Perhaps you suddenly start locking the bathroom door when you take a shower, choosing clothes that hide your body shape, or sleeping in pajamas even though you enjoy sleeping naked.

If you are single and would like to meet someone, the traces of a disease can make you feel reserved and shy or cause you to completely refrain from even trying. It used to be very taboo to talk about cancer, probably because the disease was almost always synonymous with a death sentence. Fortunately, that is no longer the case. Many people are completely cured and even more live for a long time with cancer. There are support groups and communities on the Internet, so all in all, openness has increased.

Still, having survived cancer is rarely the first card you want to play when you entering a new relationship.

With regard to sex, it is of course particularly difficult if there are scars or changes of the genitals or breasts. Every woman is aware of her breasts, how much they mean to her identity as a woman and the erotic messages they send. Even with breast conserving cancer surgery, many women feel uncomfortable about showing their naked body to a partner, or about their partner touching their breasts. Self-esteem, a positive relationship with one's own body and the ability to enjoy sex are closely linked, and the more upset a woman is about her appearance after surgery for breast cancer, the more it curbs her desire.

It tends to get better as time and life pass and the disease becomes more distant. The partner plays a crucial role here. A woman who is allowed to feel that she is still attractive and lovely will quickly rediscover the same joy of sex she felt before the disease.

Chemotherapy spreads throughout the body and affects all kinds of tissues. There are many different types of chemotherapy and the treatment can be more or less demanding, but there are almost always some side effects that affect your sex drive, such as nausea and a general feeling of being unwell and anything but sexy. You may lose your hair, not only on your head but all over your body. Your weight and body shape may change as well.

Certain types of chemotherapy stop the production of testosterone, and that means a lot, especially for men who will lose the desire for sex as well as their ability to become excited and get an erection. For a woman who has not yet been through the menopause, there is a risk that the ovaries will be damaged by the chemo and rendered unable to produce estrogen, at least for a period. This will make the mucous membranes of the vagina more delicate, making sex painful. It can feel like the vagina is too tight and too dry and increase the risk of infection.

Radiation therapy is a local treatment aimed directly at the diseased area. If you receive radiation in the genital area, it will almost always have a negative effect on your sex life, at least temporarily. Radiation destroys cancer cells, but it also affects healthy cells in the vicinity. For instance, it can destroy the cells that produce pubic hair, which may disappear completely or partially. Nerves and blood vessels can also be damaged, sensation changed and the tissue can become more rigid and drier than before.

For men it can become more difficult to get an erection. Women may feel that the vagina doesn't become wet anymore, and that it's sore, tight and easily irritated. In some cases, the vagina shortens and loses its elasticity, and it may have a tendency to develop labial adhesions or agglutination, which makes intercourse painful.

During a course of radiation therapy near the vagina, it is important to keep the vagina open, either by having intercourse if you like and can handle it, or by using a dildo that you lubricate well and insert into the vagina. Dildos come in many different shapes and sizes, and there are also many different types of lubricants. It's a good idea to get started as early as possible, as it is much easier to prevent adhesions in the vagina than to remove them once they have developed. In addition, estrogen therapy in the vagina and a good lube for sex are indispensable aids.

Heart and Blood Vessels

The most important disease of the heart and blood vessels is atherosclerosis or clogging of the arteries, which has a variety of causes. Obesity, smoking, lack of exercise, diabetes, too much cholesterol in the blood and stress are all well-known lifestyle factors. Fatty material and calcium stick to the inner wall of the arteries, which become stiff and narrow, forcing the heart to pump harder in order to keep the oxygenated blood circulating to the various parts of the body. The result is high blood pressure, which strains the heart in the long run, and the organs may suffer from lack of oxygen.

There is a risk that the blood vessels close completely due to calcification. When this happens in the heart it's called a heart attack. The high pressure can also cause the inelastic blood vessels to burst, and when this happens in the brain, it's called a cerebral hemorrhage or stroke.

The penis contains erectile tissue, three spongy tubes that fill with blood to make the penis stiff and ready for penetration. For an erection to take place, the vessels that lead blood to the penis must open and well-functioning. If they are too narrow, not enough blood reaches the penis and the erection becomes insufficient. The result is a flaccid penis, and the condition is called erectile dysfunction or impotence.

Atherosclerosis affects women in the same way, reducing blood flow to the clitoris, vagina and labia during sex. This can make it more difficult to become excited, and it can take longer for the mucous membranes to become moist.

Furthermore, some of the medication commonly prescribed for the treatment of cardiovascular disease can reduce the sex drive and reduce the flow of blood to the penis and vagina. The same applies to medication that lowers cholesterol, beta-blockers, diuretics and digoxin.

If you have suffered a heart attack or a stroke, your sex life can be impaired for a lot of reasons. Your medication may have some of the blame; however the most common problem is a fear that it's dangerous to have sex, and that the physical effort associated with sex might increases the risk of a new attack. In some cases, a heart attack causes so much damage to the heart that you must avoid sex, but normally there is no danger from being sexually active if you are healthy enough to climb a flight of stairs or do light housework.

How strenuous is sex, then? Well, the amount of physical activity associated with sex is actually quite small, unless you really work at it. Normally, it only equals very light exercise. But this can also be hard if you're not used to it. Exercise should be something you do on a regular basis. If the interval between your training sessions is too long, the risk of injury increases, and it's exactly the same with sex. The deaths that occur during sexual activity predominantly hit the untrained who do not have a regular sex life.

Sex can actually be really useful as part of the rehabilitation process after a stroke or heart attack, as it provides an adequate amount of exercise, has an overall stress-relieving effect and generally makes one see life in a brighter light.

Anyone who has been admitted to the hospital due to a heart attack, stroke or some other cardiovascular disease should receive information about sex when they are discharged. Whether one can proceed as usual or must take special precautions and if so, for how long. However, this communication is shockingly rare. It's difficult to say whether it's due to modesty, misplaced consideration or lack of imagination. So for now, patients need to take matters into their own hands and ask, and hopefully over time the attitudes of doctors and nurses will change.

Chronic Obstructive Pulmonary Disease

Chronic obstructive pulmonary disease (COPD) or emphysema is an irritation of the lungs causing them to lose some of their elasticity. At the same time, the lining of the smallest air passages become swollen, so the airflow is obstructed and it becomes more difficult to breathe. All this means that you cough up phlegm, especially in the morning, that you lose your breath easier and are more prone to catching respiratory infections.

The shortness of breath can be very pronounced, making it difficult to do everyday tasks, such as getting dressed or standing up and walking from one chair to another, and oxygen therapy may become necessary.

The predominant cause of COPD is smoking, and while a couple decades ago it was typically an old man's disease, this is no longer so. The disease strikes more and more women and can be seen in people who are not much older than 40.

It's extremely uncomfortable not to be able to get enough air, and this naturally affects the pleasure of sex. When it's hard to breathe, it's uncomfortable or even impossible to kiss or give oral sex. In addition, you live with a chronic lack of oxygen, and besides feeling like you're in really bad shape, it can also affect potency. The lack of oxygen causes erectile dysfunction, and it becomes difficult to be physically active during sex. Moreover, the treatment of COPD often includes corticosteroids, which diminishes the sex drive, and the desire is also adversely affected by the anxiety and depression that affect many with COPD.

As a COPD patient you will have to adjust to the situation in many ways. Sex will have to be as physically undemanding as possible. You will want to try out different positions to find one that is not too strenuous for your breathing, and your partner will have to be the one that is most active. In addition, many COPD patients feel that their condition is better at certain times of the day, and those hours may be the best for sex.

Incontinence and Prolapse

Incontinence is the involuntary release of urine or, more rarely, stools and gas. It is a widespread problem that can affect both men and women, but in a sexual context it is predominantly a female problem. The condition has a major influence on sexuality, because most people think a leaky bladder is terribly embarrassing. If you are afraid of involuntary release of urine or gas during the sex act and concentrate on tightening your pelvic floor muscles, you won't be able to relax and have a good time. The more excited you get, the greater the risk that you are going to leak. It can be so bad that you do everything possible to avoid such intimate situations.

There are several causes of incontinence in connection with sex. The muscles of the pelvic floor may be weakened by age or childbirth, or there may be repercussions of surgery or radiation therapy. Women with a slightly weak sphincter may also experience urine leakage when the penis hits the front wall of the vagina, and thus the bladder. And then there are some that relax so much when they have an orgasm that the body completely forgets to keep things inside.

If you suffer from incontinence and feel that weak pelvic floor muscles are the cause, the first thing to do is to strengthen the muscles with Kegel exercises. It is also a good idea to see your doctor for a check-up. There are causes for incontinence that can't be dealt with Kegel exercises, and there may be other and better treatment options.

Surgery may be an option if you have a hard time controlling your bladder and Kegel exercises don't help. Your options will depend on the cause of incontinence.

If you feel that incontinence is affecting your sex life, you need to talk to your partner about it. Your partner may not think it's such a big deal. Moreover, it is possible by simple means to alleviate the problem so that it no longer bothers you: You can use a protective cover on your bed, remember to empty your bladder before having sex and have a towel nearby to absorb the urine.

Women who suffer from incontinence may also have a vaginal prolapse, but the two conditions are not always present at the same time. Prolapse is a condition caused by lax or torn connective tissue and muscles around the vagina and is provoked by such activities as childbirth, chronic coughing and repeated heavy lifting. The vaginal walls bulge inwardly into the vagina together with the rectum or bladder. The woman may find that intercourse is difficult because the prolapse is a mechanical hindrance and blocks the vaginal opening.

But sex is made more troublesome in other ways too: It can be painful because the mucous membranes become dry and irritated, and it can be less satisfying because lax vaginal walls make it difficult to feel the movements of the penis. Some women experience accumulation of air in the vagina and feel very embarrassed by this. A mild prolapse may be cured by Kegel exercises, but more severe cases can only be corrected by an operation or a device that holds the vaginal wall in place. This will alleviate the symptoms in most women.

Obesity

A very large proportion of the population in the western world weighs too much. Many are obese or very obese, and in Europe, the proportion of obese people has doubled in 25 years. It's even worse in the United States, and obesity figures are rising all over the world as people move from the country to the cities, change their dietary habits and get jobs that don't imply physical work. From a global perspective this situation is getting worse and worse.

Being too fat impairs your sex life on many different levels. A survey of European men with an average age of 60 showed a clear link between obesity, decreased sex drive and erectile dysfunction. Obese men also had a generally poor quality of life. They felt tired, lacked energy and had low self-esteem. The link was even more apparent when sex and quality of life were correlated to their waist circumference.

A large waist measurement indicates that fat is located inside the abdomen between the intestines, instead of subcutaneously, e.g. beneath the skin. While subcutaneous fat keeps you warm and smoothes out wrinkles, the intra-abdominal fat is linked to diabetes, arteriosclerosis and hormonal imbalance. In men, this means decreased levels of testosterone in the blood. Research has also shown that obese men don't have sexual thoughts and fantasies as often as others, that their sex drive is diminished and that it takes them longer time to become sexually aroused.

In the study of European men mentioned above, even those who were not obese were at risk of having problems if their waist circumference was over 102 centimeters or 40 inches.

Women have the same problems if they are very overweight, and generally people who weigh too much have a less active sex life than people of normal weight. There may be many reasons for this, and lack of self-esteem is probably one of them. It all depends on how society views obesity, and in our western culture of abundance this is generally not considered attractive. However, in the parts of the world where being big is a sign of wealth, like some places in Africa, obese people may be more sexually attractive than slender people.

Depression

Depression is the opposite of happiness and affects how all facets of life are experienced. Nothing brings you real joy anymore, you can't find any meaning in life or your existence and you may feel it would be easiest just to end things. Energy and initiative disappear, and it is impossible to imagine bright and happy moments in the future. You cut yourself off from other people, can't bear to be social or have contact with friends and may feel that you don't love your partner anymore. Everything loses its color, the world is gray and heavy, and life is literally a nuisance.

The signs of depression in elderly people can be anxiety, agitation and unexplained physical pain, and it can be difficult to see that depression is the underlying cause.

It's not clear what actually happens in the brain to provoke a depression, but it is clear that there are changes in the brain's neurotransmitters, which are the substances that pass on messages from one nerve cell to another. These changes also affect a person's sex drive, which often disappears completely. A depressed person has neither the energy nor the interest to initiate sex, she doesn't react to erotic stimuli and she may be unable to become aroused and have an orgasm. In addition, most types of antidepressants reduce sexual drive.

If you have a partner, depression can place serious stress on the relationship in several ways. The depressed person can sink so deeply into herself that her partner feels there's no longer any contact. Just talking about things can become too difficult, and so there is a basis for misunderstandings. Lene describes her own depression like this:

> "I've been depressed for about a year now and unfortunately it's really hard on my relationship with my husband. We had a very good sex life before, but after I got sick, I'm just not interested in sex anymore. Once in a while I agree to have sex to please him and because he is my husband, but it's almost worse than nothing, because he can tell that I don't get anything out of it and he thinks that it's his fault. That he didn't do it well enough, or that I don't care about him anymore. And it makes me even more upset."

If your lover is suffering from depression, you may have to be prepared to put your sex life on hold for a while. But even someone who has no energy for sex, talking or any form of social interaction still likes to feel another person's warmth. Sitting or lying close without saying very much is perhaps the best way to show your love to your depressed partner.

Prostate

The prostate gland is located just below the man's bladder, around the upper part of the urethra. The prostate often becomes enlarged in older men, and this narrows the urethra and may cause problems with urination. The typical symptoms are frequent urination both day and night, difficulty starting to urinate and also problems emptying the bladder completely.

An enlarged prostate is a benign condition, and although it can be very troublesome, it isn't dangerous and therefore does not require treatment as long as the man is able to urinate. If the prostate becomes so enlarged that he's unable to urinate at all, there are both medical and surgical treatment options. Both can have an impact on his sex life.

An operation for an enlarged prostate does not affect a man's sexual desire or ability to get an erection, but after the surgery the man will often ejaculate into the bladder instead of out through the penis. This is not dangerous, and the next time he urinates, the sperm will simply be washed out. But it can make ejaculation a different experience than before surgery.

The medical treatment available works by causing the prostate to shrink, making urination easier, at least for a while. Some of the medications on the market may have side effects, such as low libido and impotence.

Cancer of the prostate is the most common form of cancer in men, but it often develops slowly, and many men live with a small cancerous growth of the prostate without ever noticing it. The symptoms that may come resemble benign prostate enlargement, so it may be necessary to take a biopsy in order to determine whether the condition is benign or not. Even if it is cancer, however, treatment is not always necessary, if the tumor is small and doesn't grow.

If some kind of intervention is needed, the possibilities are surgery, radiation, hormones or a combination the three. Impotence used to be common after surgery, but nowadays, if the tumor is not too big, it's possible to perform surgery in a way that spares the nerves to the penis so the man can still have erections afterwards.

Radiation therapy is tougher, and about half of men who receive it become impotent. Finally, radiation is often combined with hormone therapy that counteracts the production of testosterone. As a result, the man will lose the desire for sex, he will no longer be able to get an erection, and he may also experience hot flashes.

If you have a prostate condition that requires treatment, it will likely affect your sex life, at least for a period of time. It is therefore important to talk with your partner and your doctor about this before treatment. There may be several different treatments to choose from with varying impact on your sex life, and this can influence which treatment you choose.

When the treatment is completed, follow-up and counseling are important, also with regard to sex. This should be provided by doctors and nurses as a natural part of the information to patients, but unfortunately that's not always the case. You may need some help getting your sex life going again, and it has been shown that extended treatment with tadalafil (brand name: Cialis) helps restore sexual function after treatment for prostate cancer.

You should not wait too long to initiate treatment. The longer you wait, the more difficult it becomes. As long as you initiate rehabilitation quickly, are patient and have a loving and understanding partner, there is a good chance that your sex life will get back on track after treatment.

Diabetes

Unlike the sex hormones, the hormone insulin is vital, and the inability to produce insulin is a life-threatening condition. It is needed to transport sugar from the blood into the cells so the cells can produce energy. People with diabetes don't have enough insulin because the pancreas is not able to produce enough insulin or the cells in the body require extra insulin to transport the sugar. The consequence is too much sugar in the blood and too little in the cells, and the cells don't function as well as they should.

The symptoms you get from this tiredness, weight-loss and extreme thirst. Another important consequence of diabetes is that there is too much fat (or lipids) in the blood. Lipids, together with calcium, get stuck on the walls of blood vessels causing them to become narrower and this impedes the free flow of blood.

There are two types of diabetes: type 1, which you can develop at any age, and type 2, which was formerly known as adult-onset diabetes because it was typically a condition found in elderly people. Age is still a risk factor, but today, young people also develop type 2 diabetes. It is by far the most common of the two types and it's caused by a lifestyle with too much food and too little exercise.

With diabetes, there is a significant risk that the small blood vessels in the erectile tissue of the penis eventually become obstructed. Impotence is three times as frequent in men with diabetes as in healthy men, and a weak erection can be the first sign of diabetes. The longer a man has had the disease, the greater the problems often become. This is especially true if he is also a smoker or if his diabetes is not properly treated and his blood sugar levels are constantly too high.

However, effective control of blood glucose can improve erection. Medical treatment of erectile dysfunction with Viagra or similar medications are often effective in diabetes cases, at least as long as the blood vessels are not too damaged. But physical activity and small amounts of alcohol also helps, and the effect lasts longer than with the pills.

Women with diabetes may also have problems with their sex life. There is a tendency to develop irritation of the genitals, itching, burning and vaginal inflammation, making sex uncomfortable. In all women, sex can lead to cystitis because bacteria get pushed up into the urethra, and this risk is increased in diabetics. This can be prevented by emptying the bladder after sex, rinsing the genital area well and if necessary lubricating the labia and the area around the vaginal opening with a protective ointment of the type used for diaper rash.

If you have had diabetes for many years, the nerves to the genitals may become damaged and the sensitivity of the penis or the clitoris may be reduced. When you don't feel touching and stimulation as well as before, it may become more difficult to get aroused. In addition, both women and men with diabetes complain of reduced sex drive. They score lower on the pleasure scale than one might expect, even when taking into account the effects of the diabetes. The reason is probably stress and the impact of reduced self-esteem and the prospects for quality of life, which are a consequence of having a chronic disease.

Vera, Age 57

I'm divorced and I have lived for six months now without a man, but I'm trying again now. I'm about to take up my relationship with a former lover. I have had a good sex life earlier. It's become a bit more difficult now because I have Parkinson's and it makes my body a bit stiff.

I don't feel as much desire as before either, maybe because of the anti-depressants I'm taking. I don't reach climax anymore when I masturbate, possibly because of the anti-Parkinson's medication. But I really hope I'll be able to with my old lover. Sex is extremely important to me.

My ex-husband had a very aggressive way of making love, there was no tenderness at all. My new lover is different. He takes his time, and it's so wonderful that he's not in a hurry. We sometimes lay together, petting and fondling, but I have not had an orgasm with him yet.

He has had problems with premature ejaculation in the past, but not anymore.

Being close is more important now than when I was younger. We lie together and cuddle; it's delightful intimacy and closeness. I would like us to grow, try Tantra and enjoy loving feelings and touching all over.

I discuss sex with my women friends. One of them has a sick husband, and it doesn't matter at all to her that they aren't able to have sex. If you don't have a man, she says, you don't feel any desire, but if there's a man, you do. Me, I miss sex, when I don't have a man.

I receive local estrogen treatments in the vagina, but I still have trouble being too dry..

My ex-husband would probably refrain from sex if he couldn't get an erection. If my new lover couldn't get it up, we could still have a sex life. The moments afterwards are very important, the feeling of belonging together. It's so important for our relationship.

I'm afraid that it will be more difficult for me to have sex when my Parkinson's gets worse. I miss having an orgasm. Unfortunately, no doctor has discussed sex with me in relation to my disease. I have tried to broach the topic myself without getting any answer.

I once worked at a residential home for elderly people where sex normally is a huge taboo. There was an old couple, over 80, who fell in love with each other. The woman told me: "And we tried that thing that was so wonderful when we were younger, but it didn't work. So now we sit in the sofa and have a glass of wine and hold hands. That's also lovely."

That's a way of being together too.

A Good Sex Life after 50

Sex adds zing to just about everything. Sex on the front page of a newspaper boosts sales figures. Crime is especially spectacular if it includes sexual aspects, and advertisements more or less openly use sex as an eye-catcher. In 2010, the Internet domain sex.com was traded for 13 million dollars.

But of course, sex is – or at least it can be - fantastic. The eroticism, flirting and desire, passion and orgasm, the closeness, warmth and intimacy with the one you love. Most also appreciate the exclusivity, because you don't have sex with just anybody. When a couple has sex with each other, they confirm and strengthen their unique relationship. They show each other confidence by daring to be close, letting go and showing facets of themselves that are secret to others.

Are there other reasons for having sex, other advantages than the positive feelings and the care for the relationship? Is it healthy? Well, according to popular articles appearing on a regular basis in magazines of all kinds and on the Internet there is no end to all the good things sex can do for you. It improves your sense of smell, calms your mind, lowers your blood pressure, strengthens your muscles and your pelvic floor, flushes out your system, supplies extra oxygen to your brain, boosts your immune system and whitens your teeth. If all this were true, healthcare expenses wouldn't be much of a problem. Unfortunately there's not much scientific support for most of these claims. There is no doubt a clear relationship between health and how often people have sex. Abundant research shows that elderly people in good health have active sex lives. However, they are active because they are healthy and not the other way around.

Being healthy simply gives you better opportunities to be active in all kinds of ways, also sexually. But is there any research supporting any health benefits of sex? Is there scientific proof that we simply feel better and perhaps even live longer? Are we going to introduce sex by prescription?

The body doesn't seem to gain much from sex. As sex is a kind of physical activity one could argue that it's good exercise. This, of course, depends on how you have sex and for how long and how much energy you put into it. Unless you just lie flat on your back and enjoy what's being done to you, having sex requires some muscular work, and maybe some muscles that you don't use very much in any other situation get a little exercise. You also get your pulse up and your lungs properly aired.

But honestly - if you need exercise, you should choose some other kind of activity that is effective for your whole body and also ensures that you boost your general fitness and endurance. And if your goal is to lose weight, you would have to have a fairly unreasonable amount of sex to burn enough calories to make it noticeable on the scales.

When it comes to the soul, however, that's a completely different matter. There's the immediate satisfaction and pleasure of an erotic experience. As mentioned before, you normally don't feel like having sex with someone you don't like, so sex is a means of confirming a good relationship. The physical closeness opens the mind to the partner and sex may become a meeting point where other aspects of the relationship may be discussed. A good sex life is an indicator of a happy couple.

But the soul and mind also benefit in other ways from close physical contact with other living beings. Humans are social creatures who need contact and intimacy with others, and if we don't get it, our health can suffer. Small children who grow up without physical or emotional contact with others don't develop normal minds and social skills. Women in warm and loving relationships with their partners, who give them lots of hugs, have lower blood pressure than women who lack positive physical contact. And when faced with challenging problems, they do not become as easily stressed.

Positive physical contact improves our chances for a long and healthy life, just like understanding, empathy and support from a partner. There are many stories about elderly couples, where when one partner dies, and the other quickly deteriorates and dies shortly after. This is not a coincidence; it's quite possible to die from loneliness and grief. If you lose your partner after a long and good life together, you have an increased risk of dying in the following months.

Elderly people normally live quieter lives than when they were young: The children have moved out; working life is running smoothly or given up altogether. They know themselves and their partner; they know what turns them on and what they don't like. Their aim is normally not as many orgasms as possible within the shortest possible time, but enjoying the long, sensual path to climax. Of course, as described in the preceding chapter, there may be more stones on the road to a good sex life when you're not quite young anymore. However, there's no reason to be resigned to your fate and put up with problems that can be helped, and in this chapter we'll take a closer look at solutions and possibilities.

Checking Your Lifestyle

Good health is a sound basis for a rewarding sex life. The longer we live, the greater the differences between us become, depending on our genetic material, the environment we have lived in and, most importantly, the way we have treated ourselves over the years.

Our genes are given and basically unchangeable, and they are, in part, responsible for our reaction to influences from the environment, making us more or less resistant to negative forces. If you have inherited your mother's red hair, you're more prone than others to develop a melanoma due to sensitivity to the sun. If your father was an alcoholic, you may be at risk of becoming dependent on alcohol yourself.

There's not much to do about the genetically determined risk factors, but we can control our lifestyle and stay out of the sun or refrain from drinking alcohol. The problem is that the negative consequences of bad habits and lifestyle develop many years after we have exposed ourselves to them, which makes it difficult to motivate people to change.

An extremely potent 22-year-old man who sits in front of his computer all day, smokes a pack a day and eats a bucket of fries for dinner in front of the TV will have a high risk of developing type 2 diabetes and being impotent by the time he's 45. But that doesn't feel relevant to him, as long as he's young and believes himself immortal.

A person's sex life is actually a very good indicator of his general health in both body and mind. As long as that's working, things are not all bad. But what can you do, if you feel that both your desire and potency have begun to decline?

Well, first of all, it's a good idea to have a look at your lifestyle and focus on the usual suspects that steal health and years of your life: tobacco, overweight, stress and a sedentary lifestyle. Expose yourself to one of them, and you're in danger - together, they are a deadly cocktail. They all increase the risk of arteriosclerosis, and this will affect your sex life.

Even in men under the age of 40 there's a correlation between the amount of exercise they get, their ability to have an erection and orgasm and their general satisfaction with their sex life.

The good news is that alcohol doesn't seem to damage your sex life, at least not as long as you don't overdo it. Alcohol, especially red wine, has for some years had a reputation for being beneficial for the heart and blood vessels, and it also seems to have a positive effect on sexual performance. It may even improve the ability to have an erection - but only when consumed in small amounts. Almost every man has probably been in the situation that he set out to have a great evening with fun and drinking followed up by a fantastic night in the sack, only to find that his performance was embarrassingly poor.

So what can you do if you've become a slightly tubby coach potato with a penis that refuses to get hard? Is it too late to change your lifestyle and become a hot and virile first lover?

No, it's not. Men who start exercising and lose weight can to a large extent re-establish their ability to have an erection. Losing weight alone has a positive effect. Gastric bypass surgery can restore both the desire for sex and the erectile capacity of a man. Not only do his testosterone levels rise after the operation, but his self-confidence will also improve as his refection in the mirror changes. Women will also experience a better sex life after bariatric surgery.

For both sexes, there's a lot of good sex to gain from being physically active. Exercise is of fundamental importance for keeping hormone levels and the metabolism healthy. New research actually shows that with a proper amount of exercise, both women and men can avoid the general decline in testosterone levels that sets in for most people at the age of 20. Research has also shown beyond any doubt that exercise has positive effects on the brain. It gives you more energy, strengthens your ability to register and process signals from your surroundings and improves your memory. So exercise is a really good investment for anybody who wants to avoid disease and disorders when they get older. And who doesn't want to do that?

Talking to Each Other

If you have had the same partner for a long time, and your sex life has always been good and satisfying for both, there is a good chance that it will stay this way without much talk or discussion. But if disease or something else comes in and changes the situation, it is advisable to take it up as soon as one of the parties feels it as a problem to avoid misunderstandings, unfulfilled longings and desires or imbalance between you. Dialogue promotes understanding, and you can't expect your partner to be able to read your mind and know all your dreams, even though you may have known each other for a lifetime.

There are two important prerequisites for your conversation to bring you forward. The first is that you are honest with yourself and take your own needs seriously. You have as much right as anyone else to feel the way you do and to want things to be a certain way. Remember that sex should be a pleasure, not a duty.

So you have to make yourself clear about how you want your sex life to be. How important is it to you? Do you honestly wish to preserve it? Maybe it's simply a relief for you that it is over. Perhaps you think it's nice to go to bed in peace and quiet, read a book, with no demands to show desire and be a sexual partner. Or maybe you want to keep your sex life, but only under certain conditions. Maybe changes are needed for it to function well. In any case, it's important that you make this clear to yourself.

The second prerequisite is that you are honest to each other; otherwise your conversation will be no more than pretense. Maybe it's perfectly okay to you both that the eroticism between you has subsided. Satisfaction with sexual life may well mean that you do not have sex and that you are content with this situation.

But if it's not okay, the way forward is for you to go into more detail about things. It can be difficult if you are not accustomed to talking about sex with each other. You will have to go out of your way to get things started. You need to find the right words, make sure that you have plenty of time and that the setting and the atmosphere suit the conversation topic.

If can be a good idea if the person taking the initiative notices the partner, and if you agree on a date in advance. Maybe you want a glass of wine to help everyone relax, let go of inhibitions and shyness. You might want to sit in semi-darkness with lit candles and soft music, or perhaps it's easiest for you to talk together when you go for a walk.

Start by talking about what you each think your sex life has been like. What have you especially appreciated? In what way have things changed compared to the past? What was good before, what was not so good and what is better now? Which ingredients in your erotic life do you want to preserve? What do each of you like and dislike with regard to touching, how quick or slow things should go, are there new things that you would want to try? What turns you on, what stimulates you and what turns you off? What do you like to do to each other - to give and to receive?

Perhaps your conversations will turn old patterns completely upside down. This process requires that you respect each other and that you give each other space. The American psychologist Bernie Zilbergeld, who wrote the book *Better than Ever* about the sex lives of middle-aged and older people, divided the elderly into Lovers and non-Lovers, depending on whether they indicated that their sex life was good or unsatisfactory. He described the differences between the two groups in the following way:

> "Where the Lovers accept their partners as they are, the non-Lovers complain, judge, and try to change their partners. Where the Lovers talk about sex, the non-Lovers stay silent. Whereas Lovers are open to reality and change, the non-Lovers are closed and insist that things have to be just so. The result is ordinary or disappointing sex rather than extraordinary sex, or no sex at all."

It is vital to call attention to the importance of having a fairly regular sex life, of continuing to sense and respond to erotic stimuli. Much can be said about nature - it may not be merciful, loving, good or necessarily beautiful, but it is rational and does not waste resources. Systems that are not used are quickly shut down.

If, for example, you are weightless in space for a period of time and you don't have to use your muscles to keep your body upright, your muscles will atrophy and you will become osteoporotic. If you bury your sex life for a long time, desire can be hard to re-awaken, not so much in the younger years but when you grow older. We are certain that we will always be able to ride a bike once we've learned how, but if we don't do it for a number of years, we may feel a bit off-balance when we try it again.

The elderly, who have maintained a good sex life, or perhaps have achieved one late in their lives, work hard at it. They know that it does not come by itself; they make the extra effort because they want to keep each other, their lives together and their sexuality. They give each other time and space, see and appreciate each other's positive aspects and ignore the negative, and they nurture their togetherness in many different areas. They like each other and feel comfortable and fully accepted by the other. They can talk openly with each other about their sex life, as they can talk about everything else.

This does not mean that they tell each other everything. Respect and love naturally means that you don't want to hurt each other.

Talking to Your Doctor

A 74-year-old woman said to her doctor at the end of a consultation: "... and then there is this thing with my husband - his potency is not very good anymore..."
The doctor: "Yes, but then he is also an older gentleman."

Doctors often find it difficult to talk to their patients about sex, and this applies particularly to older patients. In the little example above, the doctor's message to the patient is that she can't really expect anything else at her age, and the patient will probably feel embarrassed about having brought the matter up. It is a difficult subject for both parties because of shyness, modesty and fear of offending the other.

For doctors, it is particularly difficult to raise the issue if there is a big age difference between them and their patient and if the doctor and patient have different genders, different religions or cultures or possibly even different sexual orientations. An American study of the extent to which gynecologists discussed sexual problems with their patients showed that women did so more often than men, and younger gynecologists did so more often than older ones.

Sexuality and the way you practice it is something very personal, with private experiences you rarely talk openly about with friends and acquaintances. You are familiar with the way you do it, but not with the ways of others. Doctors may think it feels awkward or may be afraid of offending the patient by talking about things that are too private, but this is an unfounded fear. Most seniors are actually happy to discuss sexual problems with their doctor. If they get sick, they want to know whether the disease will affect their sexual desire or function, and they also want to know whether the medicines they are prescribed or the treatment they need will affect their erotic lives.

And this is where the doctor's next concern may come to view. In the words of a group of British doctors, is it a fear of opening "Pandora's box". That all of a sudden there will be problems swarming around that the doctor is neither trained to solve nor has the time to address in sufficient detail in the short time available for a consultation.

But there is just no way around it – doctors must overcome their reluctance to discuss their patients' sexuality for several reasons. For one, there is the growing awareness that sexuality is essential for human life and that it also applies to the older generations, which are increasing in size. But it's not just about quality of life. There are also hard-core medical facts, which it is important to disclose. If your sex life suddenly deteriorates, it may be an early warning of a medical problem that your doctor should hear about and possibly treat.

As mentioned, there's a clear link between erectile dysfunction and cardiovascular disease. And because the blood vessels in the penis are so small compared to, for example, the coronary arteries of the heart, a man may suffer from erectile dysfunction for up to five years before he displays other symptoms of atherosclerosis. In 60-year-old men who have not had any heart symptoms but consulted their doctor regarding erection problems, 75 percent have high cholesterol, 25 percent have diabetes and 25 percent have hypertension. Erectile dysfunction may therefore be an early warning that it is time to do something if you want to avoid cardiovascular problems for the rest of your life.

Talking to a Sex Therapist

If there are problems you can't solve yourselves, and your own doctor is unable to help, it can be a really good idea to see a sex therapist. Although there may be a good explanation for your problems, such as a chronic illness, which you have to accept and live with, a sexologist can give you advice on how to achieve the best possible sex life under the given circumstances.

It may be reassuring to know in advance that a consultation only comprises counseling and talking. A sexologist does not perform treatments, such as touching the client. And clients will not have to take their clothes off during the consultation.

A clinical sexologist or sex therapist is trained to deal with such problems as lack of desire or arousal, orgasm problems, premature ejaculation and anxiety, shame and guilt that prevent people from fully enjoying their sexuality. It is important to choose a sexologist with care. In most countries, this area is not regulated and does not require authorization. Anyone can call themselves a sexologist and take people into treatment without any other qualification than their own personal experience. If you want to find a sex therapist, you should ask your doctor or search the web, but remember to be careful and ask for qualifications and references.

Strengthening Your Pelvic Floor

The pelvic floor is a group of muscles and ligaments that keeps you together at the bottom, so to speak, and ensures that your intestines, bladder and other organs stay in place when you stand upright. The pelvic floor is like a hammock attached to the pubic bone in front and the tailbone at the back. The rectum, urethra and vagina pass through holes in the pelvic floor.

The rectum and urethra are normally closed by muscles called sphincters, which relax when you pass urine or stools and which you should be able to tighten and squeeze together to control bowel movements and urination. The vagina has no sphincter but a muscular tube surrounding it. Just like any other muscle, the pelvic floor tends to become weaker with age, and there are also other factors that affect it: obesity, prolonged coughing, pregnancies and heavy lifting strain the pelvic floor and make it even more important to maintain it and keep it in shape.

It is important for both men and women to learn pelvic floor exercises, also called Kegel exercises. So how do you do them? Well, provided that the nerves of the pelvic floor are not damaged, the muscles can be trained like any other muscle. But if you look for a machine in the gym to train your pelvic floor muscle, you won't find it and you will find yourself left to your own efforts. The great advantage with this is that you can actually train anytime and anywhere without others noticing it.

To begin with, you must find the right muscles. This is done by squeezing around the rectum. If you are completely untrained, it's easiest to do this while lying on your back with your knees bent. When you squeeze hard enough, the rest of the pelvic floor will follow. It should feel like your anus moves upward in the pelvis when you squeeze. Try not to use the muscles in the buttocks, tummy or thighs, and you must not push or hold your breath while you squeeze, as this will put strain on the pelvic floor instead of strengthening it.

If you are in doubt whether you are doing it right, you can put a finger lightly against the anus and feel the sphincter tightening. When a man squeezes right, he will feel the base of the penis moving up slightly, and women can feel with a finger in the vagina that the muscles contract and the upper part of the vagina becomes elevated. Once you've got the technique down, you can proceed with the training. Just go ahead and squeeze as much as you can. A muscle will only become stronger if you make it work a little more than it is actually capable of. So you need to slowly increase the squeeze until you are up to the maximum you can handle and then squeeze just a little more; hold it as long as you can, then hold it a little longer, preferably ten seconds. Then release the squeeze slowly and gradually. Squeeze again and repeat it a few times. Do this a few times a day. Once a day, you should also do a series of rapid squeezes where you only squeeze for a second, but still with as much strength as possible.

The result depends on the effort, and there are no shortcuts. But as with other training the result makes it worthwhile. A stronger pelvic floor means better sphincter control and less risk that you will leak urine, gas or stools, also during sex. This makes it easier to relax and enjoy. When you build muscle, new blood vessels are formed to supply the muscles with the oxygen and nutrients they need. This means that the exercises also increase blood flow in the pelvis, which will make it easier for you to become excited, get an erection or become wet in the vagina.

For a woman, a stronger pelvic floor also enables her to use her muscles to play with the penis during intercourse and improve sensation. When it comes to men, the effect of pelvic floor exercises has been studied after surgery for prostate cancer, and it's been noted to improve the ability to control urination and bring more sexual satisfaction. While there is little research on how pelvic floor muscle training (PFMT) effects older people's sex lives when there are no problems with incontinence or otherwise, it's hard to imagine that they can do any harm, so just go ahead and squeeze.

Improving Your Erection

What makes a man masculine? According to a Swedish study, in men's own eyes, it's confidence, the ability to have sexual intercourse and independence. The Swedes felt that impotence or erectile dysfunction was a more devastating blow to masculinity than being unemployed, but in Scandinavia there is considerably easier access to help for men who lose their jobs than for men who become impotent.

A man who loses the ability to get an erection and complete sexual intercourse will be hit hard in his self-esteem and self-confidence. He will apologize, explain away, withdraw from situations that can result in sex - but out of embarrassment, he will rarely seek help. And a lot of men have problems with erection, some only occasionally, others regularly. One-fifth of all men suffer from erectile dysfunction.

The problem becomes more frequent with increasing age, and almost one in three men over the age of 65 can no longer get an erection sufficient for sexual intercourse.

In this respect it's a little easier for women. Intercourse may be uncomfortable and it may hurt, but it's pretty rare that women simply cannot follow through. Also, since femininity is not associated with being sexually assertive in the same way as masculinity is, women are not hit quite as hard in their self-image if they can't have sex.

Previously it was thought that most cases of impotence have a psychological cause, and this may also be true for very young men. But now it has been shown that one can actually detect a physical cause in four out of five men with erectile dysfunction. The most common cause is atherosclerosis.

When Viagra came on the market, it was a huge help to elderly men with erectile problems. It was in many ways a revolution, both culturally - elderly people suddenly "had a right" to a sex life - and of course medically. Until that time, the general perception as we know was that erectile dysfunction was due to psychological problems that should be treated with psychotherapy, a treatment that was largely unsuccessful as most cases were due to hardening of the arteries.

But Viagra affected the blood vessels in the penis so a formerly impotent man could get an erection and also keep it long enough to satisfy himself and his partner. A precondition for Viagra and similar preparations is that the man is sexually aroused, so it's ineffective if he has lost interest in sex.

Wanting sex starts a cascade of events, which not only get the man thinking about sex and perhaps - depending on the circumstances - taking action to have it, but also make his body ready for it.

In cases of severe atherosclerosis, the blood vessels can be so rigid that they are unable to dilate. As a result, there is a limit to how much effect you can expect from Viagra. But for many men, especially elderly men, the problem is that they do not have enough of the substance that enables dilatation of blood vessels during the erection, thus increasing blood flow. This substance is called cGMP, and Viagra works by ensuring that there is enough cGMP in the blood vessel walls.

The sum of the whole process will be a penis that becomes rigid and stays rigid for a longer period of time. Typically, the effect of Viagra sets in 30-45 minutes after you've taken the pill, and the effect lasts for four to five hours. There are a few other substances which act in much the same way as Viagra, for example Cialis. However, with Cialis the effect is longer, up to 36 hours.

All medicines carry the risk of side effects, and this is also true of potency-enhancing products. The expansion of the blood vessels is not limited to the penis, but also affects other parts of the body. Some men will turn red in the face, while others have headaches. Blood pressure may fall as well. Furthermore, certain medications, such as nitroglycerin used to treat angina, should not be used at the same time as Viagra.

In addition, Viagra can temporarily affect vision, so blue and green colors seem different or everything has a bluish tint.

Viagra has no effect on women. It does not increase their desire, lust, ability to have an orgasm or orgasmic quality. But erectile dysfunction is not just a problem that affects men, it also indirectly affects their partner and their relationship. The partner can see that the man has less desire than before and withdraws from sex life, and female partners of impotent men report that they themselves have problems with reduced sexual desire, vaginal dryness and having an orgasm.

Psychologist and sexologist Julia Heiman, from the Kinsey Institute, and her colleagues studied the effect of treatment with potency enhancers on a well-established relationship between a man with erectile dysfunction and a woman without sexual problems. The men were given Viagra, and this improved their ability to get an erection as well as increasing the number of successful and satisfactory intercourses. The men felt generally more satisfied sexually, but their emotional well-being also improved.

Their female partners also felt that their sex lives improved. They were not only sexually satisfied more often, but they also felt more sexually attractive and found that their desire was stronger.

Before the men in Julia Heiman's study were treated with Viagra, their female partners felt sexually dissatisfied, and they seemed to believe that their sex life with their spouse was gradually collapsing. They wanted a change and they were looking for a solution to their men's erectile dysfunction. But this is not necessarily the case for all women. If you are getting up in years and your sexual desire has gradually subsided, it may feel natural that sex is no longer a part of life. If so, Viagra can bring more trouble than joy.

The American sociologist Annie Potts has interviewed 27 women whose men started taking Viagra. The women were on average 53 years old and had not had sexual intercourse for some years. The aim was to investigate the negative consequences of the use of Viagra, and Annie Potts revealed several problems. The attending physicians generally considered erectile dysfunction as an exclusively male problem, and the women felt that they had not been consulted in the process. The men saw the doctor alone and initiated treatment without discussing it with their partners, who were apparently supposed to be happy and satisfied with the result.

But a postmenopausal woman who has not had intercourse for a few years does not necessarily think that it is so great to be approached for sex, sometimes several times a day. Her desire may have faded, and her body is not prepared for or used to having sex. She might experience tears in the vaginal mucosa, vaginal inflammation, cystitis and pelvic pain.

But even if the woman doesn't really want to have sex, it's not always easy to just say no. The woman may want to support her husband and his re-emerging masculinity. She wants to give him the good experience of successful sexual intercourse. And now that he has taken this rather costly pill and proudly exhibits a huge erection, of course it should be used; the investment should generate a return, so to speak.

Some women in Potts' study reported that sex with Viagra had become much more focused on the penis, and this was no improvement. Suddenly it was all about the man's erection and his orgasm, while the women missed the caresses, seduction and foreplay. These things were not as necessary anymore, and it was a drawback, particularly for older women who needed a longer foreplay to make the vagina moist and ready for sex.

There were also women who thought it was okay that sex was no longer part of their lives. They didn't miss it, considering it part of the natural aging process, and they had no trouble living with things the way they were. There were other things that kept them together with their partners, such as love, friendship, a shared history and common values. They felt that sex for them was a closed chapter, and they did not think there was any reason to reopen it. On the contrary, they could feel bulldozed by their men, who, with their new desire and ability to perform sexually, were suddenly in a very different place than the women were themselves.

In this way, treatment with Viagra and similar drugs can contribute to causing a distance between the parties in a relationship. This is a good illustration of how important it is to talk with your partner about your expectations to the relationship, including your sex life.

Viagra and similar preparations are first-choice medications for impotence. If there's no effect, there are other possible solutions. For instance, there is a preparation that can be injected directly into the penis 5-15 minutes before the man wants to have sex, and a pellet containing a Viagra-like substance to put into the urethra. There are also mechanical devices like a rubber ring to put around the base of the penis to help it stay erect for a longer period of time, and the penis pump, which helps create erection by using a vacuum so the penis fills with blood.

Hormones – Yes or No?

As I have said earlier, there are a myriad of hormones with various functions in our bodies, but when it comes to their influence on your sex life, estrogen and testosterone seem to be the most important, which is logical enough as they are mainly produced in the ovaries and testicles. Estrogen fluctuates a lot during a woman's lifetime and has very different levels in the blood during the menstrual cycle, pregnancy and breast-feeding. When menopause comes, it decreases abruptly. This usually does not directly affect the woman's sex drive. Generally, it is a fact that women who have had a good and pleasurable sex life before menopause continue to enjoy it after menopause. Decreased sexual desire depends more on the state of your health, your relationship to your partner and satisfaction with life in general.

Lack of libido cannot be treated with estrogen. But low estrogen levels after menopause can still wreak havoc in your sex life, because the lining of the vagina becomes thinner and loses its elasticity and moisture. This means that the mucosa is more likely to develop small tears in connection with sex, which is painful and makes it easier for bacteria and inflammation to take hold. In fact, thin and dry mucous membranes are the main reason why post-menopausal women abstain from sex.

If you want to keep the vaginal mucosa the way they were before menopause, there is only one thing that really helps – estrogen. Estrogen comes in many different forms: as tablets, suppositories, patches, vaginal inserts, implants, cream and gel. Not all varieties are available in all countries.

Normally, your doctor will prescribe local vaginal treatment if the only problem is a tender and dry mucosa. If there are other symptoms of discomfort, such as hot flashes, vaginal treatment won't be enough and the woman may want tablets, patches or gel.
Estrogen treatment comes with both risks and benefits, which vary with the woman's individual health profile. So a good talk with your doctor is important before initiating treatment.

It is also important to use a good lubricant when you have sex. The best ones contain silicone, they don't dry out on the skin as quickly as the water-based products tend to do, but remain effective for several hours. You can usually buy these products in a pharmacy, but as there is not much privacy some may feel too embarrassed to go there.

A store selling sex toys will often be a much better option. Here you get professional and friendly advice, not just about good lubricants, but also about many other interesting things that can be used to spice up your sex life. If you can't bring yourself to enter a store like that, there are plenty of possibilities to buy these products online.

Treatment with estrogen is only an option for women. With testosterone, the principal male sex hormone, it's another matter. As previously mentioned, it is a hormone that can boost both libido and stamina for both men and women. But a man needs to have a blood testosterone level that is abnormally low for a testosterone supplement to be effective. If the man's testosterone levels are normal for his age, his sex drive will not be improved by taking more. He may only experience the quite unpleasant side effects: heightened anger and aggressiveness, greasy skin and acne and an enlarged prostate.

Women may find that a testosterone supplement has a positive effect on their sex drive, particularly when they grow older. In many countries it is actually common to treat post-menopausal women with hormone supplements containing both estrogen and testosterone. Testosterone seems to have a good effect on the libido, arousal and satisfaction in women, and it can also increase a woman's energy and overall well-being. But it is important to note here that when researchers perform studies on medication for low libido, there is always a very large placebo effect. This means patients who without knowing it receive inactive calcium tablets instead of testosterone, still notice an effect of the medication – because they believe that the pills contain something that makes them tremendously horny.

In fact, some claim that sex is actually something that goes on far more between your ears than between your legs, and this doesn't seem all that far-fetched.

Another important thing worth noting is that testosterone also can have side effects for women. It may increase unwanted hair growth and acne, and some may also suffer hair loss. However, compared to the benefits, many women feel that they can live with these side effects.

Other possible risks are more significant: testosterone may increase the risk of atherosclerosis and hypertension and may have unwanted effects on the metabolism, causing fat to build up in the abdomen. The importance of these changes is not yet clear and as with estrogen, it probably depends on the dosage and the risk profile of the individual woman. Uncertainty about estrogen supplements for women has caused some countries to withdraw medications that were once permitted and in Denmark there are no testosterone preparations at all intended for women.

Finding a New Friend

Imagine yourself at the age of ten. It's May and the sunlight is seeping through the bright green trees and in through the classroom windows. The teacher is trying with all his might to keep your and your classmates' attention focused on the German cities. You feel a small tap on your shoulder, and a little paper ball lands on your desk in front of you. It is a crumpled corner from an exercise book, and it says: "Do you want to go out? Pick one: Yes, No, Maybe".

Fortunately, you can fall in love regardless of your age. And even if you aren't lucky enough to meet the love of your life, it's great to have a good friend to share experiences and thoughts with. But friends come and go, and sometimes you want to meet somebody new.

There have never been as many people over the age of 60 who been divorced and remarried as there are now. So what do you do if you want to find a new friend who might also become a lover? If there don't seem to be any candidates among your closest acquaintances, and you don't have the energy to start any new hobbies or join any more clubs, then you look online.

Young people have been dating online for a long time, and the elderly are also growing more and more comfortable with it. Many may feel some resistance the first time the idea pops up. Do you really have to offer yourself like that when what you really want is to be discovered and seduced? Is it not dangerous and overpopulated with charlatans with sinister intentions looking to get their hands on your money? Won't people be able to recognize you on the street and whisper behind your back: "Have you seen his profile on Senior Dating? He isn't that good looking in real life, is he?"

Well, nothing ventured, nothing gained. Start by carefully considering what you really want to achieve by looking for a partner online. Do you want a good friend, are you looking for a steady relationship or just somebody to have sex with? Somebody you share interests with? Or do you want new inspiration? Do you want to get married and share a home and future? Of course you can change your mind along the way if you meet someone who is just right (or wrong), but it's a good idea to think through the possibilities before embarking on the project.

On American dating sites you will primarily see the classical sexual patterns, and when it comes to the older generation it's probably the same in Scandinavia. Men are normally looking for a woman who is younger, and women often want a man who is slightly older than themselves. However, women over 75 prefer a younger partner.

Older women often date with a slightly different purpose than older men. Men who become alone are more eager than women to find a new partner and are more likely to want to marry. Women are more reserved and explain this in part by the fact that they generally have a good life with friends and family. They are not interested in losing their independence or having to take care of a man who is really only looking for a cook and a housekeeper. They are looking for a new partner as someone they can go out and have fun with, talk to about things other than what women talk about, and someone they can travel with. Sex is an option, but not a requirement, and by and large they may be searching for another type of man than when they were young and looking to get married and have children.

Once you have reflected on what it really is you want, you need to find the right forum. There are lots of dating sites with different names and purposes. Some are for sex, others for people with a certain type of education or of a certain age. Ask somebody who has tried it and surf the Internet until you find a place that you think looks good for you.

Now that you have found the right site, it's time to create your profile. It's not always easy. You will want to write a presentation of yourself that's not too long, but that still contains the information that will attract the right type of person and make the wrong ones stay away. So it's about finding the right balance between boldness and modesty. Be honest about yourself and what you want, because you could wind up attracting the wrong people. And be original and personal, if you can. It may well be that the things you appreciate most in life are cozy domesticity and walks in nature, but this is rather non-specific and won't really help you look like the special person you are.

It's a good idea to ask someone who knows you well to help you highlight your attractive qualities. There is no need to mention the negative ones. Use more text to describe who you are than who you are looking for. Remember that it is important to provide potential partners with the information that makes them want to meet you in particular.

American research has shown that men and women write different things when presenting themselves in contact ads. Women describe their appearance, and men typically highlight things that give them status. Men also place emphasis on appearance when choosing a date, but there doesn't appear to be a specific age when women stop being attractive to men. However, it depends on how old the man is. More than half of men over the age of 50 find women attractive no matter how old they are.

In the beginning, you will want to pay a lot of intention to the wording of your ad. As you become used to the fact that you have actually put a personal ad online, you may grow bolder and experiment with changing it, be more personal and reveal more about yourself in your profile. Most people become less reserved and dare to write a little more as they become familiar with the process. Also, if you've had a couple of contacts that you feel weren't right, you may want to take stock of this and change your ad accordingly.

Be anonymous in the beginning if you feel that's the safest thing. Never give away your real name or other personal data from the outset. If you really want to be private, you can create a separate email address that you only use for your personal ad.

It can be a good idea to talk on the phone before you meet. If you don't want to disclose your phone number you can buy a prepaid card for your phone and use it when talking to someone you don't know yet. And when you are going to meet for the first time, start with a cup of coffee on neutral ground, that is, somewhere in public where there are plenty of people. There is no need to be too picky about who you meet for coffee, people may very well have qualities that do not appear in writing, and if you don't think there's good chemistry between you, it's okay to politely say no to further meetings right away. Those are the rules of the game. But take care not to let your expectations get too high and expect love at first sight. What you want at first is just to meet somebody new, to expand your circle of acquaintances and then see what it leads to.

If you're lucky, flirting is the next step. And here I'm sure you don't need my advice! You will soon discover that it is just as fun as when you were younger. Perhaps even more fun, because now you have a better understanding of who you are and how to play the game, and can enjoy it for what it is and secretly endorse the other party for their elegant moves.

So good luck - I leave you with the words of the French actress Jeanne Moreau, who said:

> "Age does not protect you from love. But love, to some extent, protects you from age."

Ingemarie, Age 64

I was married for 30 years, and I was 55 when we got divorced. And our sex life... well, it was really quite boring, for the last 15 years at least. I didn't feel that he wanted me at all. I had breast cancer and had an operation and became menopausal, and he just couldn't handle that. That was huge loss for me. He didn't want to admit it, but once he just blurted out that he didn't like my body anymore and found me disfigured. That was really painful.

Well, over time that marriage just got worse, and I was really relieved when it ended. I hadn't had sex for years really and I didn't miss it, never suddenly felt the desire, you know. Of course I thought that my life wasn't over, that some other man might turn up eventually, so I'd better keep it up a little and so I masturbated from time to time. When I got turned on, it was fine, great; I could have two or three orgasms in a row.

And then when I was 59, I met Jorgen, a widower who was a little older than me. Some friends introduced us and we began going to the movies and having dinner and so on, and finally we became lovers.

And you bet we were both nervous the first time we went to bed together. One of his friends had given him a Viagra pill he could take if the situation became critical... And I was extremely shy and didn't want him to see me naked, so I had to do all sorts of strange dodges to get into bed. It worked out all right, and he didn't have to take the pill, but it wasn't, well ...

Really, it's become much better since then! We make love several times a week now. We have ordinary intercourse and quite often kiss and lick each other. Both of us like that a lot. You tend to get sore more easily down there at our age, and it's a bit gentler to use your mouth, you know.

I think sex has changed for the better as I have become older. It's not so frenzied; there is more foreplay and more cuddling afterwards too. It's relaxed and easy. We spend a lot more time on the sexual act now than we did when we were young.

I have learned that orgasm will come, if you just give yourself time. It doesn't have to be rushed through; foreplay can take all evening. He uses Cialis now and then to get hard, but not when we're on holiday. He doesn't have to use it then. So I'm absolutely sure that it's stress that sometimes makes it difficult for him to get an erection.

Acknowledgement

My intention with this book is to convey the facts about sexuality in
older age. The scientific data is taken from peer-reviewed articles in
international literature, mostly found through the database
MEDLINE. Added to these facts are my own interpretations and
subjective views, which inevitably, to a large extent, reflect the
culture I live in. You, the reader, will surely have your own views,
and if you disagree with mine, I hope that, at the very least you will
find our differences of opinion and attitude intriguing.

I want to thank the people I have interviwed for this book; they have
told me the most intimate details of their life., and I am grateful for
the confidence they have demonstrated in me. I also want to thank
my husband Povl Christian Henningsen. Without the inspiration,
support, and coffee he brought me at the right times, this book
would never had been written.

www.ingramcontent.com/pod-product-compliance
Lightning Source LLC
Chambersburg PA
CBHW060907280326
41934CB00007B/1220